Dr Nick Fuller is a leading obesity ı
worked in both corporate and acade
position he is responsible for the clinical research program at the
Boden Institute, located within the Charles Perkins Centre at the
University of Sydney. He has helped thousands of people at all
stages of life with their weight-loss and lifestyle journeys over the
past 15 years and investigated a broad range of treatments, including diet and exercise programs, appetite hormones, commercial
programs, complementary and conventional medicines, medical
devices and surgical treatments. He has degrees in exercise physiology, nutrition and dietetics, and a doctorate in obesity and weight
management. For more information visit intervalweightloss.com.au
or the 'Dr Nick Fuller's Interval Weight Loss' Facebook page.

interval WEIGHT LOSS LOSS for women

Dr Nick Fuller

PENGUIN LIFE

AN IMPRINT OF

PENGUIN BOOKS

PENGUIN LIFE

UK | USA | Canada | Ireland | Australia
India | New Zealand | South Africa | China

Penguin Life is part of the Penguin Random House group of companies whose addresses can be found at global.penguinrandomhouse.com.

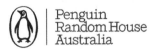

Penguin
Random House
Australia

First published by Penguin Life in 2020

Cover photograph by Acharaporn Kamornboonyarush/EyeEm via Getty Images
Cover design by Penguin Design Department © Penguin Random House Australia Pty Ltd
Author photograph courtesy of the University of Sydney
Typeset in 12.5/17 Adobe Garamond Pro by Midland Typesetters, Australia
Printed and bound in Australia by Griffin Press, part of Ovato, an accredited
ISO AS/NZS 14001 Environmental Management Systems printer

 A catalogue record for this
book is available from the
NATIONAL
LIBRARY   National Library of Australia
OF AUSTRALIA

ISBN 978 0 14379 109 6
penguin.com.au

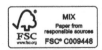

As with all my books, this is for you, Dad. You inspired me to always read and write, to convey my work into words, and to teach and help others. Not a day goes by that I don't miss you. You will be forever in my thoughts.

CONTENTS

INTRODUCTION

You have a problem. It's why you're reading this book. In fact, most of us have a problem. A problem that can be caused by two things – food addiction and dieting. You can't stop eating your favourite foods and you can't put an end to the battle with your weight. The binge and deprivation cycle is common to many women, and it's why you are battling your weight at every turn. But I'm here to tell you – it's not your fault, and you're not alone.

To begin, we must look at our ancestors, whose origins are ultimately the cause of our contemporary problem. We evolved to seek out calorie-rich foods and our body learnt to protect itself by shutting down and storing fat when food was scarce – like in the time of hunting and gathering. This was needed in order to survive. But that environment of our ancestors was completely different to what we see today. Compare desperately seeking out food for days, sometimes weeks, then having a feast to last until the next round, to today's abundance of tasty, calorie-rich foods – they are everywhere, and we have a hard time resisting our urges to have just one chip, just one almond croissant, just one serve of bacon on the side of our breakfast. Scientists call it an evolutionary mismatch – once-useful traits needed for survival are, in our modern-day environment, now harmful. Hence, this inability to resist isn't a lack of willpower – it's because of our biology. Our body will always work to protect its current weight (its 'set point', which we will discuss in detail through the book), and this defence mechanism is now causing a big part of our collective weight issues.

This isn't just a problem for women, it's even worse for men. The prevalence of excess weight and obesity is heavily skewed towards men (75 per cent of Aussie men are overweight or obese, as opposed to 60 per cent of women). However, this reality isn't reflected by how women (and men) see themselves, nor by the weight-loss industry's attitudes towards who exactly needs to lose weight and the uptake of diets in women versus the uptake in men. Women are the first to admit they have an issue. Think of your friend/ sister/mother/partner complaining about how she, a woman in a perfectly healthy weight range, needs to lose weight. Studies have shown that women are significantly more likely to consider themselves overweight than men and subsequently are more likely to do something about it. That's good news – sort of. The problem is, women turn to diets, and as I have learnt from extensive research, this has serious consequences, none of them good.

A recent survey from the United Kingdom showed that by the age of 45 most women will have tried 61 diets, attempting four to five diets every year. Over a lifetime, they will have spent an average of 31 frustrating years of their life on a diet. Madness. Ever since the 1980s, all we have been talking about is diets. Diets, pills, buzzwords, shakes, late-night TV merchandising and magic calorie potions pop up every day of the week. Today, it's 'health' influencers online. These very clever marketing examples promise the quick results and miracle cures we are after. But it hasn't worked, and it never will. Because of diets, we are dealing with a huge public health challenge with serious psychological and physical ramifications. Diets have not made us thinner; they have only contributed to the very problem they proclaim to solve. Whenever you impose a caloric restriction on the body it will go into shutdown mode. It will ensure you regain all the weight you lost, plus a little extra as a safety net. This was crucial for our ancestors' existence, in order to survive.

This reality is especially confronting for women, a great many of whom start on a diet despite not having a weight problem. Which leads us to another significant social issue we have created for ourselves. We have normalised a faulty, dangerous thought that women in a healthy weight range are overweight. It runs through every thread of social media, every TV ad, every Hollywood sex scene and every magazine cover. This faulty thought has distorted what is factually normal. It has turned a physical phenomenon into a psychological phenomenon and devalued any woman who isn't a photoshopped Instagram model. This issue is only compounded when you consider a woman in her mid-to-later years of life – it further validates her lack of self-worth and renders those impossible standards even more futile, particularly when her weight has been a major factor in her low self-esteem and lack of confidence throughout life.

This creates a further challenge for health professionals like me. Not only are we battling a diet industry full of misleading and wrong information – and therefore fighting what feels like a losing battle to get the right intel out there – we are also fighting that skewed perception of what is normal. Telling women in a healthy weight range that they are overweight leads to confusion and fear and doubt. It also leads to big corporations in the diet and 'wellness' industry lining their already ample pockets with your hard-earned money.

From my perspective as a qualified expert in this space, what I overwhelmingly see is a need for a total overhaul of most people's approach to weight loss. In this book, I will focus on the female attachment to weight and provide solutions to weight problems by outlining the six habits of successful long-term weight loss (the six principles of the Interval Weight Loss (IWL) plan). I will also address the common weight gain following pregnancy and menopause – two of the biggest challenges a woman will face over her lifetime.

Whatever your reason for starting on a destructive diet cycle – unrealistic social expectations, a parent who told you to lose weight in high school, a cruel comment from a boyfriend long ago or a genuine need to lose excess weight – the important thing is that by picking up this book, you are rejecting that negative approach to your body. You have started your IWL journey – a lifelong strategy for safely and progressively changing your body's set point and maintaining a weight you are comfortable with, for life.

Just as the problem is evolutionary, the solution is evolutionary too. And this is the point of difference between diets and the evidence-based IWL plan. Since our body's evolutionary response to dieting – what it perceives to be a food scarcity – is to become heavier, the IWL plan taps into the body's evolutionary adaptive ability to become lighter through cyclical weight loss. The IWL plan allows you to lose a set amount of weight every second month with imposed 'breaks' – periods of weight maintenance – every other month, thus enabling you to redefine your body's 'set point' at intervals along the way. This allows you to achieve a weight loss that your body doesn't fight against, so you can keep it off. And unlike a diet, it won't have you scouring the supermarket for obscure ingredients, counting calories, cooking for hours, weighing ingredients, following set meal plans, depriving yourself of food or completing an unrealistic and militant exercise program. In fact, the IWL plan is the opposite: it gets to the bottom of the real issues you need help with. You will learn how to manage your favourite comfort foods, not demonise them. Your relationship with food will improve, as will, I hope, your relationship with yourself.

Whatever your reason for picking up this book, it is the first step to lifelong change. Scientists have shown that 66 is the magic number of days it takes to ditch a bad habit – so, your first 66 days will be the hardest, but it's worth it, I promise. Come on, let's get started!

PART 1

CHAPTER 1

BIOLOGY IS BLOCKING YOUR SUCCESS

How often have you heard someone say: 'It's easy – you need to eat less and move more!' This piece of advice dates back as far as Hippocrates in the fourth century BC, and not much has changed since. Diets are based on this very foundation and despite their different approaches, they are all essentially the same. They set a caloric restriction and develop a set of arbitrary rules to create a fear of certain foods, to ensure you consume less. But whenever you restrict the number of calories you eat, powerful biological forces come into play to fight the resulting weight loss. This leads me to the underlying reason why we as healthcare professionals treat obesity as a disease. Would you consult with an unqualified person if you had cancer? A broken leg? Diabetes? Heart disease? Why is it any different if you have obesity? It shouldn't be. The increasingly saturated digital 'wellness' space is overrun by thin women spruiking laxative tea or muscle-bound men telling their millions of Instagram followers it's easy to get a six-pack with just one weird trick. As you probably know by now, those people pushing their pseudoscience diets and 'wellness' plans are only making your problem worse. There is no evidence behind their claims. A before and after shot is not science and certainly doesn't tell the whole story – especially what that newly svelte person looks like in six months' time.

Despite your best intentions and significant financial outlay, following that advice or program won't help you lose weight in the long term, and it especially won't help with the contest of two of the biggest challenges a woman will face during her lifetime: conception and menopause.

Your lack of long-term weight-loss success has never been due to a failure of willpower; it is due to your biology. During our time as hunter–gatherers our body became very efficient at conserving energy and storing fat, going into shut-down mode by lowering its metabolic rate: the amount of energy burnt at rest. This would prevent the body from losing large amounts of weight so it could maintain a body weight with relative stability over long periods of time – necessary when you didn't know when your next meal would come, not so necessary now.

Scarcity of food also meant that our ancestors sought calorie-rich, nutrient-dense foods, which offered the best bang for buck – a crucial advantage when calories were hard to come by. The same is not true in the modern-day environment. The desires that were extremely helpful to our ancestors get us in considerable trouble today. Basically, the same urge that saved our forebears from starving to death is what is making it so hard for you to now resist the cheese before dinner . . . and the chocolate after.

Nowadays, you don't have to walk more than a couple of steps before you stumble across a vending machine or corner shop. Our favourite foods are everywhere and we have a very hard time resisting them because we are programmed to want them. Unable to resist, our waistlines grow. In response, women turn to diets, which are heavily marketed towards them. Women think they are fat, the diet industry encourages them to think they are fat, and consequently far more women than men embark on what will ultimately be a futile foray into dieting.

Many diets have stemmed from the 1970s Atkins revolution, which proclaimed that carbohydrates are the devil and the thing making us fat. But even though most modern diets were invented from this time onwards, obesity rates have trebled. Diets have done nothing to curb the obesity epidemic – indeed, they have contributed to the very thing they claim to diminish. Today's diets do more harm than good. This is especially confronting for women, a great many of whom start on a diet despite never having a weight problem.

The problem with dieting

Dieting is one of the biggest stresses you can impose on your body. Other examples include physical force, surgery or a heart attack – pretty scary stuff. When you impose a stress such as dieting, it will trigger a cascade of events within your body to protect itself. I will elaborate on these shortly.

There are two main reasons diets don't work. First, they are unrealistic and unsustainable, requiring us to omit certain foods or even entire food groups. We are unable to stick to them for very long because of that biological imperative to eat and eat, and after we come off the diet or program we reintroduce the foods, go back to our old ways and stack the weight back on. Second, we are all tuned to a 'set point', which our body protects, and no diet or weight-loss program addresses that. What's more, a lot of these diets are dangerous for our long-term health.

But, *some* diets work, don't they?

When it comes to weight-loss success, you will always have the one-percenters who succeed on a particular diet or plan, and that's fantastic for your cousin's girlfriend or your friend's colleague who just won't stop talking about their victory on the latest diet. This doesn't mean the diet works. Individual responses to diets vary enormously, and, regrettably, the biological imperative to protect our current body weight means most of us are set up to fail before we even begin. People won't hesitate to tell you of their short-term success, but rarely are they still bragging down the track. This is particularly relevant for those trying to conceive. Obesity is one of the biggest causes of infertility, and in a desperate attempt to conceive, many women opt for the quick fix of rapidly dropping weight to fall pregnant. If you go on a diet with the goal of falling pregnant, you *may* succeed – though many do not – but as a consequence you will struggle with your weight in the long term for the very reasons you will learn about in this chapter. Your body's ability to defend itself against weight loss will also mean you will end up heavier with each subsequent pregnancy.

What is the Interval Weight Loss plan?

The IWL plan is not a diet, nor is it a temporary fix for a long-term problem. Therefore, there are no exclusions and no forced inclusions with the IWL plan, because these only lead to you craving a food you have omitted, hating the new exercise you have started, or abandoning the hobby you have taken up.

The IWL plan involves the following:

- A month-on, month-off plan following the principles of the IWL plan so you can recalibrate your body's set point, reach your body's optimum weight, and stay there.
- Lifestyle changes to achieve the goal weight loss of two kilograms in the weight-loss months, interspersed with weight maintenance months.
- Learning how to retrain your brain so you reduce your addiction to processed and fast food.

- Eating more wholesome, nutritious foods that are filling and tasty, allowing you to eat more than you're used to.
- Enjoying five meals per day and following the tunnel plan of big to small portions throughout the day (breakfast as your biggest meal and dinner as your smallest).
- Applying the 10-minute rule before going back for seconds so you learn how to tune into your appetite-signalling system and know how much to eat.
- The freedom to relax and enjoy more treats and takeaway foods during the weight-maintenance months (to allow your body to get used to its new set point).
- The flexibility to customise the plan to fit your lifestyle choices and include dietary restrictions; for example, vegetarianism, coeliac disease, type 2 diabetes or dairy intolerance.
- Learning how to improve your sleep quality.
- Exercise that you enjoy and can fit within the constraints of your lifestyle.
- Additional support and a more guided approach by signing up to the Interval Weight Loss online program.

It does not involve the following.
- Depriving yourself of food.
- Calorie counting or following set meal plans.
- Weighing out portions of food for each meal.
- Complex cooking that requires you to track down an abundance of ingredients for each meal.
- Locating obscure ingredients in supermarkets or health-food stores.
- Cutting out any foods or alcohol (unless you're pregnant or breastfeeding).
- Food waste using impractical ingredients.

- Adopting an exercise or activity routine that is not sustainable or enjoyable.

What is the 'set point'?

My own research, as well as that of other renowned and qualified experts across the globe has proven that we all have a 'set point'. This is the weight our body protects – the weight it feels most comfortable at, and it is the underlying foundation of why the IWL plan works – because it works *with* your body, rather than against it. If you have been gaining weight over a long period, your set point is likely to be the weight you are currently at (possibly the highest weight you have ever been); unless you are still regaining weight from a recent diet attempt. This varies enormously from person to person. For you it might be 78 kilograms, for the person next to you it might be 94 kilograms, and for Pat down the road it might be 124 kilograms.

Recall how the hunter–gatherer was very good at lowering its metabolism when food wasn't available. Well, this was their body protecting the set point, to ensure their weight stayed stable over time. In fact, our body protects the set point whenever a stress is imposed on it. And one of the biggest stresses on the body is dieting. When you follow a diet, your body starts to function differently; it thinks it is going to be starved for a long time and so holds on tight to where it is now, its set point, otherwise known as your starting weight. Unfortunately, this means your body is hardwired to prevent you from succeeding. Worse still, the body is extremely clever and will prepare itself for any future bouts of starvation or dieting you impose, by keeping a little extra in reserve. You end up worse off for going on the diet. The best way to visualise this is by comparing two people of the same starting weight, body composition and characteristics. When you follow them up over 10 years, the person who has been dieting will be heavier than the person who did nothing about their weight. Hard to comprehend, isn't it? This research comes from a fascinating study that followed more than 2000 sets of twins over 10 years – a twin who had dieted just once was twice as likely to gain weight as the non-dieting twin, and this weight gain increased with additional dieting attempts.

How does the body protect the 'set point'?

When we go on a diet, our body compensates by changing several key biological pathways. At least eight different biological protections kick into gear with dieting, which predispose a person to regain any weight they lose. In fact, the stress imposed on the body from a diet has unfavourable effects on a myriad of mechanisms regulating our behaviour and weight.

1. Metabolism

Your metabolic rate is how much energy you burn at rest. It is determined by how much muscle and fat you carry. As muscle is more metabolically active than fat (i.e. it burns more energy than fat), a person with a higher muscle mass will have a faster metabolic rate than someone of the same body weight with a higher fat mass. With weight loss, as expected, your metabolism will decrease because your body mass decreases (and you typically lose weight from both fat and muscle stores). We can account for this expected decrease in metabolism by putting numbers into some fancy calculations. However, the scary thing is, even after crunching the numbers, there is a decrease in your metabolism by a further 15 per cent beyond that which can be accounted for by a reduction in body mass. This means for every diet you attempt, the rate at which you burn off your food slows down significantly. Our research has also shown that often a person's metabolism won't recover from dieting, and it will be slower than before they started, even after they have regained all the weight. A well-researched example of this comes from contestants who appeared on the TV show *The Biggest Loser*. Following up with the contestants six years after the program, not only had the majority stacked the weight back on, but they were burning fewer calories every day than before their stint on the show. Prior to going on the show, they burned on average 2610 calories per day, which dropped to 2000 calories at the end of the show. But even after regaining most of the weight six years later, their metabolism had further slowed to 1900 calories per day. So, when you lose weight your metabolism slows by 15 per cent in order to defend your set point. Worse still, it may not recover if you continue to impose stress on the body with diet after diet.

2. Energy source

While you are resting and reading my book right now, your body is predominantly burning its fat stores. This is a favourable state, because burning fat uses more calories than burning carbohydrates. However, when you lose weight, your body will start to work differently and shift the type of energy source you use, from fat to carbohydrates, to ensure your body holds onto its fat stores. This ensures you burn less energy at rest and consequently you start to regain the weight you lost. This is yet another of your body's biological defence mechanisms that kick into gear to protect its set point. Very clever, isn't it?

3. Appetite hormones

Your appetite hormones play a large part in ensuring your day-to-day weight stays stable. This is thanks to hormones produced in the gut and fat (adipose) tissue telling your brain when and how much to eat. For example, when you are hungry, one such appetite hormone released from the stomach called ghrelin will light up a part of the brain called the hypothalamus telling you to eat. And when it's time to stop eating, several other hormones are released from both the gut and fat tissue to signal your brain to stop eating. But when you lose weight these appetite hormones will change their function to promote weight regain by telling you to eat more, and will suppress your feeling of fullness. So, the ones that warn us we need to eat will rise and the hormones that suppress our hunger will dwindle. Put simply, your body begs you to gorge when you deprive it of food. And again, this goes back to evolution and the history of humankind. They ate to survive and went hungry for long stretches. Our DNA harbours a fear of starvation and will protect against this situation. But worse still, just like the frightening change in metabolism that you witness when you lose weight, a similar shift occurs in your appetite hormones. That is, even after you have regained the weight you lost, your appetite hormones do not return to the same levels they were before dieting. They remain out of balance even after regaining the weight, which means you continue to feel hungry even after stacking the kilos back on. You will end up bigger than before you started.

4. Autonomic nervous system

Another of the biological protections previously preventing you from succeeding on your weight-loss journey relates to your autonomic nervous system. The autonomic nervous system is a control system that regulates body functions such as heart rate and breathing rate. It is made up of the sympathetic and parasympathetic nervous system. The sympathetic nervous system is referred to as the 'fight or flight' system, while the parasympathetic nervous system is referred to as the 'rest and digest' system. The systems work to oppose one another, whereby one will activate a physiological response and the other will inhibit. Whenever you lose weight, your body will react by shutting down, so that you burn less energy at rest. I explained how your metabolism slows when you lose weight, but it also means your heart rate and breathing rate will decrease as the parasympathetic nervous system takes control. This is your body's way of dealing with the stress by trying to eliminate it. It will slow down with dieting in order to restore its set point and regain the weight you lost.

5. Thyroid gland

The thyroid gland is the gatekeeper to your metabolism. A healthy thyroid means your metabolism is firing, and a sluggish or poorly functioning thyroid means the amount of energy you should be expending will be compromised. Under normal circumstances, your thyroid gland will produce hormones (medically known as thyroxine and 3,3',5-tri-iodothyronine – try rattling that off at the dinner table next time you're telling your friend about the science behind weight loss), but when you restrict calories or the amount of food you eat, fewer of these hormones are secreted, which ends in a reduction in the amount of energy you burn at rest. Yet another clever way your body works to protect its set point.

Everyone likes to talk about their thyroid gland when it comes to excuses relating to their weight. Thyroid issues can be problematic on your weight-loss journey, so if you're worried, go to your GP for a simple blood test that can indicate whether your thyroid is functioning normally.

6. Adrenal gland

The adrenal glands produce a range of hormones, including the stress hormone cortisol. When a stress (as with dieting) is imposed on the body, the pituitary gland stimulates the release of adreno-corticotropic hormone, which acts on the adrenal glands to produce cortisol. An excess of cortisol production leads to weight gain, and when you restrict the amount of food you eat, or lose weight, the cortisol level in your blood increases. Much like the thyroid gland, the adrenal glands also play an important role in regulating your weight and will work to protect your set point.

7. Brain function

Typically, diets tell us to restrict certain foods in order to reduce calorie intake. However, when we scan a person's brain after weight loss, we can see that restricting or cutting out certain foods or food groups in their diet results in a change in brain function. This is why you can only cut out entire foods for a limited amount of time before the desire for them comes back with vengeance. What we see is a heightened activity in the reward-system part of the brain. Simply put, your brain starts telling you that you should reach for all those foods that you have cut out and that you miss. You give in to your cravings because those foods give you pleasure, and they release the feel-good chemicals called endorphins and the learning chemical called dopamine, which remembers that feel-good response next time you see it. But that's not the full extent of it. The other significant change that a person will experience with dieting is a reduced activity in that very clever part of the brain called the hypothalamus and areas involved in the emotional control of food intake. This results in a decreased control of food intake and an impairment in the ability to sense a positive energy balance following dieting. It ends up triggering a psychological response dubbed the 'what-the-hell effect' – a vicious cycle of indulgence, followed by guilt, followed by greater indulgence. You end up eating the whole packet of Tim Tams instead of just the one. Again, more ways in which your body has been proven to defend its set point.

8. Appetite

Dieting results in not only an increase in hunger but also a change in the perceived rewarding properties of food and a preference for high-calorie food. Typically, someone who is overweight will desire foods high in fat, but after dieting, the same person will see a change towards food preferences that are high in both fat and sugar. This results in the consumption of higher calorie foods that are lower in nutrition, and consequently weight regain back to your set point.

The IWL plan is not a theory, not a fad, not the latest craze. It is not a celebrity program based on unproven anecdata or testimonials. And it is not a 28-day, six-week, eight-week, ten-week or three-month program on which you lose the weight and regain it shortly after. It is a scientific method based on years of clinical and academic research. And it is *not* intermittent fasting, or any form of fasting diet, despite the conclusions that some people jump to when they first see the title.

As mentioned earlier, fundamental to the IWL plan is the universal notion of the 'set point' and being able to overcome the well-researched biological protections you have just learnt about, to ensure you can redefine your set point without your body fighting itself. Diets impose big stresses that the body responds negatively to, whereas the IWL plan imposes small stresses at monthly intervals the body responds positively to.

Everybody has an optimum body weight, but years of stress on the body has meant that this is now a silhouette within your current figure. The IWL plan taps into your body's evolutionary desire to take it back to its natural preferred weight – its optimal weight – which allows it to be efficient in its day-to-day activities. Just imagine that within everybody there is an outline of what your body wants to be – a silhouette you will discover (or rediscover) by following this plan. This applies to everyone – you can be tall, short, male, female and any cultural heritage, it doesn't matter. It can be followed by anyone and with any amount of weight to lose. Those who have more weight to lose just need to follow the plan for longer. The capacity for change is already within you.

The *U.S. News & World Report*

I will help you redefine your current set point so you can achieve your goals; whether it be to regain control of your weight, lose weight so you can fall pregnant, prevent your weight spiralling out of control with each subsequent pregnancy, or deal with the weight-gain stresses of menopause – but you need to fully apply yourself to the IWL plan and not allow yourself to be distracted by the new celebrity diet that hits the shelves tomorrow. Remember, anyone can go out and follow a four-, eight- or 12-week program and lose some weight, only to regain it, plus interest, just as quickly.

The *U.S. News & World Report* is an annual American report that ranks diets based on nutritional balance, health benefits, ease of following, safety and weight loss. A leading group of qualified experts in the United States apply an objective scoring system to each diet to calculate an overall score. The bottom 10 from 2018's report featured the keto diet, the fast (5:2) diet, Atkins and Paleo – all the programs we so regularly see spruiked by celebrities, Instagrammers, magazines and even our well-meaning friends. For 2018, the worst one was the keto diet. In 2019 the bottom-ranked diets were again the keto diet, the fast (5:2) diet, the Atkins diet, the Paleo diet, the hormone diet and the Whole30 diet.

The reason these diets score so badly on this report is because many are unsafe to follow, put you at long-term risk of disease and they lack the science to back up their bold claims. They also don't address the one thing everyone struggles with – weight regain. People can often lose weight on these diets but they all struggle to keep it off.

The Paleo, Atkins and keto diets (and all of their anti-carb friends) all advocate the cutting of carbs. It is, however, dangerous to exclude such vital macronutrients. These diets make out that sugar, gluten, wheat and grains possess a mysterious toxicity that makes us fat, but science has proven that the inclusion of wholegrain carbs in your daily eating plan will not only help you on your weight-loss journey, but also protect you against diseases such as type 2 diabetes, heart disease and colon cancer. Eliminating carbs will help you experience short-term and rapid weight loss due to a decrease in body water, just like with any diet that is low in carbohydrate, because carbs carry a lot of water, which ends up weighing quite a bit. But there is no research to show these diets can deliver sustainable weight loss, and you end up stacking it back on – another reason they score so badly in the annual *U.S. News & World Report*.

As for diets such as intermittent fasting – which also come in many forms these days, such as 16:8 and 5:2 – they also have many fundamental flaws. For example, on the 5:2 diet you eat normally for five days of the week and cut your calories to an extremely low 25 per cent of normal intake on two non-consecutive days of the week. This equates to just 600 calories for males on the two fast days and 500 calories for females – the same number of calories as two donuts. The lack of nutritional guidance on what to eat on the five days you aren't fasting and what constitutes a healthy eating pattern raises many red flags. Different forms of intermittent fasting (16:8 and 5:2, to name a couple) are just fancy ways of cutting calories. You will see a short-term result just like with all other diets, but you will regain the weight you lose (remember, this is engrained in your biology). Intermittent fasting is no better than any other diet and hence it scores badly in the annual *U.S. News & World Report.*

It is very easy to bring out a diet with false and misleading claims, often written by people who are not qualified healthcare professionals and whose suggestions are not backed by scientific literature. Some of the companies espousing diets even have a vested interest in you not losing weight in the long term, so you go back and buy more of their four-, eight- or 12-week programs. They give you quick results to validate your success and then let you think it's all your fault when you put the weight back on.

Your task

At the end of each chapter in this book I have set you a task. Your first task is to write down on a palm card (or photocopy) the following quote from Henry Ford:

'If you always do what you've always done, you'll always get what you've always got.'

Stick this on your fridge or a wall as a reminder that you must be prepared to adopt a new way of thinking and acting as you

The typical journey for someone on a vicious dieting cycle

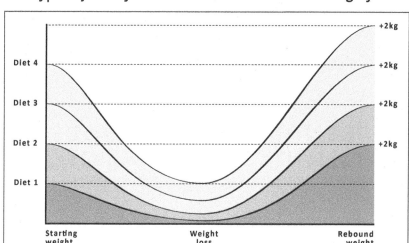

move on to the next chapter in the book. This marks the beginning of your new journey, of learning to prioritise your health and take care of yourself.

I'm not going to have you starving and skinny in a couple of months' time only to see you stack it all back on just as quickly. But I will help to make you lighter for the rest of your life, so you never have to think about diets or your weight ever again.

The IWL program is not a 'quick fix' that promises a 10 kilogram weight loss in two weeks. It will, however, result in you achieving better health and your long-term weight-loss goals – undoubtedly a good trade-off. Tiny changes will lead to bigger changes, until your life does transform and the IWL plan becomes a way of life.

CHAPTER 2

IDENTITY EXCUSES VERSUS IDENTITY ACCOUNTABILITY

Before I teach you the six principles of long-term weight-loss success, the very first step in helping you succeed on the IWL plan is to make you accountable for your actions. It's a subject I discuss with all my patients, and one I refer to as *identity excuses* versus *identity accountability*. In this chapter, I will separate *identity* and *accountability* and show how the bridge that we have built between the two is *excuses*.

To be ready for change you must first understand where you are today, so we can then discuss where you want to get to tomorrow. While this may sound simple, my experience with my patients and those in the IWL community teaches me that it is not. I refer to this as the *identity-accountability gap*.

Identity is how we think about ourselves. 'I am this, I am not that' statements. This identity becomes our story, and we spend much of our lives validating our story. 'I come from a family of [hard workers, devout Christians, staunch Labor supporters, et cetera].' You can fill the statement with whatever you like, but at the end of the day this is an identity you have created for yourself based predominantly on family, social and cultural experiences.

To an extent this is fine and normal, but when this identity gets challenged the potentially negative impacts might reveal themselves. Consequently, identity excuses repeatedly come up, and a common one relates to genes.

Debbie: 'My mother was large, as are my sisters, so it's not as easy for me as it is for other people.'

Chloe: 'Losing the weight after my second child is much harder than the first. It runs in my family.'

Many also have cultural foundations. As my workplace is in the centre of Sydney – a demographically diverse part of town – I have patients from many different cultures and backgrounds, and from a research perspective I can see that certain excuses relate to culture.

For example, Anglo-Australians have a strong affinity with unwinding over alcohol; southern Europeans have a strong affinity with unwinding over lunch and dinner feasts; and much the same can be said of Polynesians, who have a strong sense of family identity and socialising.

Michelle: 'We go out regularly for after-work drinks. I can't say no to a drink when my colleague goes to the bar.'

Janine: 'We have a large extended family and most weekends we meet up and share our traditional food over long lunches.'

There is no denying that this introduces a challenge. But again, these are just identity-excuses that are impeding the patient from achieving success. More importantly, here's what happens when these identity statements appear in my clinic: we go around in circles, with me attempting to assist the patient, and the patient building their case (through identity excuses) as to why they have never succeeded.

I do not want to appear harsh. I have total empathy for these identity excuses because I, too, have had to face my own. But the straight, hard truth is that so long as these identity excuses exist, there can never be any real sustained improvement.

This is the principal challenge for all my patients and the principal challenge for me as the practitioner. For me to be effective in helping them to enact change I must first begin with identity.

I ask: 'I want you to tell me all the reasons, no matter how silly or trivial you think they are, why you've struggled on this journey; every last one.'

Identity accountability

Let's think of some of those possible identity excuses now:

Since I've had kids, it's harder to lose weight.
I work long hours and don't have time for exercise.
I must have bad genes, because I've tried everything and can't lose the weight.
I think I have a slow metabolism, because I don't eat much but I keep putting on weight.
My hormonal changes have led to weight problems.
Kids mean I don't have time for myself.
I think I have an underactive thyroid, because I can't shift the weight.
Since going through menopause, it has been harder to lose weight.

While I don't want to disrespect any of these statements, the fact is most of us will think of any number of excuses to deflect our accountability of owning our problem. This type of thinking is deeply planted in our sense of who we are, our identity, and when we are presented with the stress of change our self-defence mechanisms immediately spring into action and revert to our identity excuses.

This is a hugely complicated topic, so I want to simplify it. If we allow ourselves to trust in the potential for change, if we put down our long-held beliefs linked to identity excuses and say, 'I'm ready to do everything that needs to be done,' then we are ready to convert identity-excuses into identity-accountability.

Here are the words that we need to repeat to ourselves: 'There is absolutely nothing that stands in the way of me taking ownership for my success.' So, with this identity accountability in mind, how would some of those previous statements now sound?

Debbie: 'My mother was large, as are my sisters, so I'm even more motivated to make this change so that they too can be inspired by what's possible.'

Chloe: 'Losing the weight after my second child has been challenging, but I will become a healthier mother for my two children and inspire my family and show them that it can be done.'

Michelle: 'We go out regularly for after-work drinks. I can still go out and have an alcoholic drink, but not six, and on occasion I can even say *no* because I have to get home.'

Janine: 'We have a large extended family, and most weekends we meet up and share our traditional food over long lunches. It's the family moments that matter most and I can still be who I want to be.'

What is required of you?

The IWL plan will equip you with truthful, research-based advice to help you succeed on your journey. But what *you* must do is much harder. You must want to, be open to, and be ready for change. You must have the courage and the honesty to break free from your existing mindset so that you learn to value the future more than the present.

You must *not* treat the IWL plan as the next diet. This is not an all-or-nothing approach. If the IWL plan starts to feel a little too much, I suspect you are still applying the all-or-nothing approach that you do when you start a diet on a Monday after an indulgent weekend of bingeing. Many of you are very knowledgeable when it comes to food and diet. And in fact, most of my patients have spent so much time researching food and exercise, you could say they pretty much have a degree in dieting. But none of those things have helped them manage their weight.

The IWL plan involves a pledge to change your life, and as I will explain in the next chapter, having weight loss as the ultimate, single goal can be completely detrimental to that. You will only end up in the weight loss = success and weight gain = failure spiral; and consequently, measuring your entire self-worth by how much you weigh on the scales. This is common with many of my patients on the weight-loss merry-go-round – our current society supports this paradigm. In the next chapter, I will help you overcome this attachment to weight.

Your task

Using the template on page 23, I want you to write down all your identity excuses. Seeing them on paper and staring you in the face is the first step to identity accountability. Rephrase each of the statements to take ownership and be accountable to yourself. Write them down on palm cards and stick them throughout your home or in a place that is highly visible. Excuses are one of the toughest challenges to overcome.

Identity excuses

*Since I've had kids, it's
harder to lose weight.*

*I work long hours and
don't have time for exercise.*

Identity accountability

*Since having kids, I make
my health a priority so that
I can be a good role model for
my children.*
*I block off time in my
calendar for exercise every day
and I partake in activities
I enjoy.*

....

....

....

....

....

....

....

....

....

....

....

....

....

CHAPTER 3

WHAT DRIVES A WOMAN TO SUCCEED?

The next step in helping you succeed on the IWL plan is to gain a better understanding of your motivations. An example that comes up often for my female patients is their wedding. Many women want to lose weight for their big day, and many succeed. Driven by the motivation to have the most exceptional day of her life, she wants to look beautiful in both real life and in the photographs that will tell the tale of that wonderful day. She is so motivated by that thought, that losing weight for the bride-to-be is a task she achieves entirely through her own willpower. This is a wonderful thing, except that after that pinnacle moment the vast majority of brides regress over a period back to their pre-wedding weight, and put on weight for years to come.

So, I ask the question: What truly is your motivation, your goal? For me, the best motivations are not the ones that focus on a moment in time, such as a wedding or a half-marathon. These are short-term motivations. The best motivations are long term, when people can describe the type of life that they envisage for themselves. One that will bring happiness to their family and a sense of fulfilment to themselves. For example, to be a better role model as a mother, to deliver a healthy baby, to set the right path for their children or to have better health. It's no surprise that one of the great motivators is a life-threatening health scare. That moment makes a person value life and appreciate what they truly have that is worth holding on to. But no one should wait until this moment. Now is the moment to look at your life and admit to yourself that you are not happy with your weight and that nothing until now has worked.

Replacing the old with the new

For you to achieve your goals, you must substitute your current behaviours with new ones. For example, if my patient is being asked to give up something to which they have a long-held attachment, they will need to replace it with something else. And the best thing to replace that with is a goal (a new behaviour) that is truly exciting and motivating. We engage in behaviours because they feel good, so if you remove one behaviour, you need to replace it with a new, positive behaviour. For example, seeing friends in a cafe setting can also be achieved by seeing friends while going for a walk. Or, the amount of time you spend on social media can be replaced by catching up with friends, so you can find out face-to-face what they have been up to.

Breaking old habits

Simply changing your daily routine and breaking daily habits will result in you achieving your goals on the IWL plan. This means doing something different every day, and it doesn't have to be food- or exercise-related, it can be anything behavioural. For example, it might be writing in a journal of a morning, driving a different way to work, helping out at your local library with community events, going to bed earlier and waking up earlier, reading on the bus instead of looking at your phone, listening to a podcast every evening or limiting your use of social media – there are apps available to help with this. When it comes to exercise, you could try walking a different route or exercising with a friend. With food, it might mean shopping at a different grocery store, shopping in a different suburb or grocery shopping online. These are just a few examples – if you change up your current daily routine with new habits, you are well and truly on the road to success.

Setting goals

When setting goals, your sole focus should not be weight loss. You will still achieve weight loss and you will still need to monitor your weight (I'll explain how to later in the book), but by no means should this be your only motivation. Instead, I want you to focus on goals and forming new positive habits, such as increasing the number of exercise days per week, reducing the number of meat-eating days per week, including vegetables on the plate with more meals per week, or reducing the number of days watching television per week.

There are four things you need to apply to each goal you set:

1. Research clearly shows that you should set goals that you can actually enjoy. This will increase your likelihood of sticking to them. If you know that you hate going to the gym or running, don't tell yourself you're going to start these activities. Instead, find a goal that is likely to have some intrinsic enjoyment or that is likely to become more enjoyable over time. It could be something as simple as going for a bike ride or a walk.

2. You need to set goals that have a range, so you feel successful even if you don't meet the magic number you have set

yourself per week. For example, instead of saying, 'I'm going to exercise every day of the week,' set yourself a target that's a range of days that you are going to exercise per week (for example, three to six days). Setting a range can be more effective than an absolute number, because one number can be unrealistic and make you feel like a failure if you don't achieve it. Revisit your goal range regularly to establish what is and isn't working, and to build it up over time until it becomes part of your daily routine.

3. With each goal, you need to make it a habit that becomes part of your daily routine. This is where automation can play a useful role. For example, when first commencing an exercise routine (for example, walking) pick the days that you are going to exercise and add it to your calendar as a meeting. If it's gym classes you prefer to attend, pre-book the classes that you like and at a time that suits you. For many it is important to do it first thing in the morning, to get the endorphins pumping and gain a sense of ownership of the day, while others love to break up their day with some structured activity in the middle. If your goal relates to spending less money on takeaway food and you want to save that $100 per week that you typically spend on eating out, automatically transfer that portion of your pay into a savings account so you can't even touch it.

4. Lastly, research has shown that writing down your motivations/intentions/goals will better help you succeed. If you write down your goals (I'm going to get you to do this at the end of the chapter) you are far more likely to achieve them when compared to just thinking about them.

Crafting your environment

The most successful people craft an environment in which temptations don't arise. For example, your goal might be to stop going to the bakery every day. Sensory cues that are associated with positive outcomes become motivational triggers. What I mean by this is, when you walk past the bakery and see the pastries and cakes in the window it can trigger an overwhelming urge to want them. Yet if you change your daily walking route so that you don't walk past the bakery, you won't experience its sensory cues and therefore it won't trigger your motivation to want them. You won't find yourself resisting the urge to eat these fattening foods. Another goal might be to reduce your frequency of checking social media. The first step would be to delete it off your phone or to log out of your account to make it harder to access. This is how you craft your environment to support the goals you have set.

Contingency plans

Of course, there are always the scenarios where you happen to find yourself in front of the bakery and in this instance, you need a contingency plan. If you struggle to walk past the shopfront and say no to the bakery treats (as many of us do), you can fight the urge to give in with a practice called *episodic future thinking*. This refers to the capacity to imagine or stimulate experiences in your mind that might occur in the future. When deciding about whether you should eat the cake, imagine yourself in the future, at an event such as your graduation, your birthday, or any sort of fun and uplifting event where you are likely to be celebrating. If you can imagine yourself at the event enjoying it, parts of the brain will light up that instinctively weight the future more heavily in the decision-making process. You will be less likely to eat the tempting foods because you value that future event. If you do happen to succumb to the little voice in your head telling you to buy that cake, it's not the end of the world, and you shouldn't beat yourself up for it. The most important thing to do in this situation is to reflect on these instances so you can establish what to do next time you encounter the same situation. By allowing yourself to still eat your favourite foods (I will teach you about this later), you will enjoy them and won't feel guilty when you walk past the store.

Partner or buddy support

We know from research on social psychology just how important relationships are. Accountability and commitment play an important role in your success. We know that when people set goals together and create an action plan for achieving them (for example, sending one another weekly updates), they are more likely to achieve the goal and continue it past the end of the formal period. This may mean discussing with your partner changes that need to be made in the household, or it might mean finding a buddy who can go on the IWL journey with you. This then becomes a commitment to one another to ensure you both adopt a healthier life. If you do choose to do this, it is important to regularly communicate on your progress. Carve out shared time – perhaps while exercising – where you can check-in together and hold one another accountable. It's also a good way to help regulate each other's goals. The small successes you make on your way to a goal may not be recognised by yourself, but your partner or friend may help point those out for you. They can also help put things in perspective if you find yourself falling off the bandwagon, by encouraging you to reflect on your progress to date.

Alleviating the burden of having to cook every meal

There are recipes at the back of this book with suggested portions, but these are only a guide and it is better to cook more food so that you, your partner or your kids have leftovers for the following day. We don't all have time to prepare all our meals from scratch every day, so utilising leftovers for lunch is a perfect way to keep you on track and prevent you eating out. The last thing we have time for in the morning is preparing meals for the day. It's hard enough getting the kids ready. Leftovers alleviate this stress and pain and keep you on track with your IWL plan.

The influence of peers

Finding an appropriate buddy can be challenging. Homophily, or the tendency to associate with others who are similar, is noteworthy, but so is the potential of friends to influence each other beyond the similarities between them. What I mean by this is, research has shown a link between social network structure and patterns of obesity, and how friends can have an influence on a person's body weight. Bearing this in mind, it may be challenging to find a friend to go on this journey with you; someone you know will support you every step of the way and not undermine your activities. The last thing you need is someone putting the banana bread in front of you at the cafe or pouring you the glass of wine without even asking. If you think this may be you, fear not, because there are people who will support your journey, and this is where the IWL community group may come in handy and be particularly relevant to you.

'IWL Community' Facebook group and online program

Following the release of my second book – *Interval Weight Loss For Life* – there were numerous requests to set up an online program for additional support and accountability while following the IWL plan. Even if you find yourself a suitable support buddy, you may also benefit from the online program and accompanying 'IWL Community' Facebook support group to check in with others following the IWL plan; people at all different stages, and people with similar experiences to you. The first couple of weeks are going to be the hardest, so learn from others along the way to better understand the plan. There is no doubt that you still need to be accountable to yourself, but someone checking in on you can also help make you accountable and can be very powerful.

What is considered a success?

The transition to what is discussed in this book may take some getting used to, but you will get used to it and you will feel better for it. Years of habits and addictions don't change overnight, but they do change. Start with small changes, because these will lead to big changes, and before you know it you will have developed new positive habits that become a way of life. This is how you should measure success. If you do this – that is, consistently change negative behaviours into positive behaviours – it will inevitably lead to your desired outcome of weight loss and improved health.

Your tasks

Task 1

Your first task for this chapter is to write a letter to yourself about what success means to you. It might just be a sentence devoting a commitment to yourself, in writing, that you wish to become a better mum, to shape a better future for your children or to lead a healthier life. Remind yourself to keep an open mind about everything I will be asking you to do.

As you write your letter, I encourage you to reflect on what I have told you in this chapter and to focus on your motivations and intentions rather than a specific goal. Your motivations are who you want to be and how you want to live. I am going to get you to list three motivations/goals. For example, instead of the goal being to lose weight (which is what most of us want to do), your intention could be to make sure you exercise 5–7 days per week; to cook at home 4–6 nights per week; and to reduce TV viewing to 3–5 days per week. Your goal will be to build each of these new healthy habits over the next month. And it can be any habits – it could be to use your phone less often or to start spending more time with family and friends.

Task 2

Your second task is to write down the goals that you have just listed in your letter. You will find a template at the end of this chapter. Make sure each goal has a range and that you have a new behaviour to replace the old behaviour. For example, your goals could be:

Goal 1: Reduce TV viewing to 3–5 days per week.
New behaviour: Build a vegetable garden and attend to it 2–4 days per week.

Goal 2: Participate in physical activity 4–6 days per week.
New behaviour: Go for a morning walk with girlfriends 4–6 days per week.

Goal 3: Reduce social media usage on the morning commute to 1–3 days per week.
New behaviour: Read a book or listen to a podcast 4–6 days per week.

You could even write these goals on a palm card that you can carry in your handbag or place on your bathroom mirror. Or you might wish to take a photo of it and use it as the background on your phone. Anywhere that's visible, to serve as a gentle daily reminder of your goals and what you are going to achieve.

Now, write your letter and your goals. You will revisit these goals each month on the IWL plan.

Goal 1:

New Behaviour:

Goal 2:

New Behaviour:

Goal 3:

New Behaviour:

CHAPTER 4

THE SIX PRINCIPLES OF THE INTERVAL WEIGHT LOSS PLAN

Now that you have a plan for making yourself accountable and setting realistic and achievable goals each month, the next step is to learn the six key principles of the IWL plan – these six habits will ensure long-term weight loss.

We know that weight loss is not just about the food we eat or the exercise we do. Obesity and weight gain are multifactorial, complex problems, and they are extremely challenging to address. Weight loss is also about how we measure success, how we prevent emotional and comfort eating, as well as how we structure and organise our day-to-day life, and simple but important things like how much sleep we get and how to let go of stressors in life. The IWL plan will equip you with all these skills and see you prioritise your health and put into action a new approach that is sustainable for the rest of your life.

The six principles

You need to carry these with you everywhere (metaphorically) and they need to become engrained in your psychology. I will briefly outline each of the six principles here and then tackle each one in-depth, in subsequent chapters.

Remember, the underlying foundation of the IWL plan is that it ensures that you overcome the biological protections and evolutionary barriers to weight loss that I discussed in the first chapter. It will also ensure you find a new passion for food, exercise and a lifestyle that you didn't think you could have.

The first principle: *You can't fight evolution*

You will impose weight-loss breaks every second month to allow your body to recalibrate at its new lowered set point along the way. This prevents your body fighting itself and ensures that it welcomes its lowered weight.

The second principle: *Reach for nature first*

You will learn how to retrain your brain to rely on nature's treats. These are foods found in their natural state, which release the same pleasure response in the brain as processed and fast food.

The third principle: *Full rainbow*

You will eat more food than you are used to with the focus on including a variety of foods and filling your plate with vegetables first. No foods are eliminated on the IWL plan.

The fourth principle: *Use chopsticks*

You will be required to sit down at the dinner table and use chopsticks of an evening because it will force you to eat more slowly. (If you are already proficient with them, this won't slow you down.

Instead, use a teaspoon.) You will also be required to make breakfast your biggest meal of the day and dinner your smallest while also ensuring you eat regularly.

The fifth principle: *Choose to move*

You will be required to seek opportunistic exercise by incorporating activity into your daily routine. You will also focus on exercise variety and getting your 'sweat on' during the weight-loss months.

The sixth principle: *No blue light after twilight*

You will be required to turn off all technology after dusk and eliminate all forms of technology from the bedroom. The evening time will be used to constructively work on your to-do list or hobbies.

What is the one thing you must do to succeed on the IWL plan?

This might seem crazy, but you must read the book *at least* three times to get a good understanding of the principles of the IWL plan. This plan must become instilled in your mind. If someone asks you what the plan is, you should be able to recite the six principles.

To succeed on this plan, it might require you to start afresh and unlearn everything you have ever been told about weight loss. The vast majority of these so-called 'experts' that you may have learnt from are unqualified and uninterested in anything but their own personal gain. You might have been misinformed by conflicting information on diet and health for years, or even decades, and it's certainly not your fault. The information you have been told is often wrong, foolish and can be downright dangerous. As we all know, anyone can claim to be an 'expert' nowadays, even our best-intentioned friends, family and colleagues, and they all love to give you their advice, especially when it comes to diet, health and wellness.

If I don't talk about it in this book, it means it's not worth worrying about. There's too much information on health and wellness these days and you would need an encyclo-paedia to cover it all. You can feel confident ignoring the magazine articles and Instagram scams about the latest and greatest – you already know not to bother, because I am giving you all the information you need. The responsibility for you to learn everything is on me, the qualified expert with decades of experience. Reading is a wonderful thing, but when it comes to the health and wellness industry, all that reading and listening to others can do more harm than good. This means: stop getting caught up on all the small things, such as whether you should be 'clean eating', activat-ing your almonds or buying organic produce, and focus on everything I'm about to tell you.

By the way, the concept of 'clean eating' means nothing – there is no such thing as 'clean' food. Activated almonds are no different to regular almonds; and whether you buy organic or non-organic is not of nutritional consequence but simply whether you choose to spend your money on it – organic food can be double the price point of conven-tional produce. Organic farmers and food producers grow food without using synthetic chemicals such as pesticides and artificial fertilisers. Despite this, organic foods are not necessarily completely chemical free – they can still use some natural pesticides, but the pesticide residues will be consid-erably lower than in conventional produce. Unfortunately, one of the biggest challenges in understanding the term 'organic' is that it means different things in different parts of the world and the regulations often change. Even packaged foods such as muesli bars can have 'organic' on their labelling but mislead you by containing both 'organic' and 'natural' ingredients. In Australia, the largest problem is the lack of regulation on the use of the word 'organic'. Anyone can slap the term on their food and you must trust the honesty and integrity of the seller. The only way to know you're buying organic is by getting a food that is 'certified organic' – these companies have paid to have their foods tested by a third party (an accredited, certified organisation).

There are far too many diets, products, foods and life-style fads these days to review or warrant discussing them all in this book. And don't worry if I don't discuss it, it's not because I've missed it, it's because it's just clever market-ing, it's not backed by evidence and it won't be of value to your success. Make notes as you go and as you re-read this book. The more you read it the easier it will come. It will prevent you resorting to old habits or getting caught up on the small things hindering your progress. This book is going to become your best friend! Trust me.

Your task

Write down the six principles of the IWL plan and stick them to your fridge to remind you of what you are achieving. Alternatively, go to the Interval Weight Loss website (intervalweightloss.com.au) and sign up to the online program for your step-by-step guide to the six principles of the IWL plan.

CHAPTER 5

CALCULATING YOUR SET POINT

In the first chapter I discussed how your body protects itself against weight loss, and the concept of our 'set point'. In this chapter I will help you calculate a goal weight loss – your new set point – so that you can overcome your biology and succeed with your long-term weight-loss goal. You will then apply the six principles of the IWL plan to ensure you achieve your new set point. And fear not, if you want the calculations to be done for you, you can sign up to the Interval Weight Loss online program from the website.

How do you know what your set point is?

Your set point is the weight that your body protects when you go on a diet and it's the weight that you will remember rebounding to each time. For many, it's likely to be what you currently weigh, if this is the heaviest you have ever been. If you haven't weighed yourself in a while, haven't been on a diet recently and your clothes have been fitting the same for a few months, you're most likely at your set point.

What if you don't know your set point?

If you don't know your current weight, your first step is to go out and buy a new set of scales and weigh yourself. This can be quite a daunting process, especially if you haven't weighed yourself in a while.

Begin by weighing yourself weekly while observing the trend in your weight over time. Do this for a month while introducing the concepts of the IWL plan (this will be your wash-out month, which I describe shortly). If your weight stays stable and your clothes have been fitting the same for a few months, you are most likely at your set point and ready to implement a weight-loss month on the IWL plan (more on this later).

If you notice your weight is increasing over the course of the month, there could be many reasons, which I will explain shortly. But if you have recently dieted and lost weight, you are possibly still regaining it. In this instance, you are not at your set point and you need to wait until your weight stabilises. The good news is you can speed up this process if you follow all the principles of the IWL plan and this will form part of your wash-out period.

It's quite refreshing to hear someone tell me they don't know their current weight, because it suggests they haven't been dieting. But there are also many people who haven't been able to face the number on the scales due to the fear that it might trigger another eating-disorder episode (which many people struggling with their weight will battle). In this instance, I suggest speaking with a close friend or therapist, so they can support you through the process. As daunting as it might sound, it is imperative that you do get this initial number and learn how to weigh yourself each week without it triggering an event. I will teach you how this can be done.

Picture Melissa, a busy mother aged thirty-five who works part-time as a TV producer while raising her three-year-old son. She desperately wants to fall pregnant again.

When I first heard from Melissa, she had recently been on the keto diet. She had enormous difficulty sticking to it and admits cheating a lot on the diet towards the end of the eight weeks. Despite this, much like all the other diets she had been on in the past, she successfully lost a lot of weight. In fact, she lost 12 kilograms over the eight weeks, but she complained of feeling lethargic and grumpy, often finding herself getting snappy at her husband, Pete. She had been off the diet for only four weeks but had already put on 4 kilograms and was beginning to panic, wondering whether she should give it another go or try the 5:2 diet she had recently heard about. When I asked Melissa what her weight had been doing over recent years, she reported that it had been going up and down for the past six years. She would lose weight, put it back on again, lose weight again, and then put it back on once more, and that it had been going up by about 3 kilograms every year for the past seven years despite all her dieting attempts. She reported being 60 kilograms in her youth, when leaving school, and then the number started to creep up during her first year at university.

Melissa went away and completed her homework. She was to read *Interval Weight Loss For Life*, she was to introduce all the principles of the IWL plan, and she was to weigh herself once a week (more on this in the next chapter) over the following four weeks, before our next chat.

The wash-out period

In order to reset your set point you will need a wash-out period to see what your weight is doing. This is particularly important if any of the following apply to you: you haven't been monitoring your weight and are unsure whether it has changed in the past year; you have an extensive history of dieting; you have recently come off a diet; you are currently on a diet. When I refer to a wash-out period I mean a period where you don't worry about what happens to your weight. Instead, your goal is to introduce all the principles of the IWL plan without being concerned if the number on your scales goes up (it's likely it will initially). The wash-out period allows your body some time to recover from previous diets and for you to start gaining a better understanding of how to implement the plan and how your body responds to it. You should not expect to switch from a diet/fad/weight-loss program to the IWL plan and get immediate results. You simply won't. It could be because you're still regaining weight from a previous diet attempt, you may have been limiting your intake of certain foods such as carbs, which carry a lot of water, or your body may have shut down from all the stress you have imposed on it previously with diets.

Reintroducing foods

Most diets require you to omit certain foods or food groups from your eating plan. In fact, every day of the week there is a new food or food group that is put in the spotlight as the cause of our weight problems. One minute it's fat, the next it's sugar, then it's carbs and now it's dairy. All too often I hear patients tell me they are avoiding certain foods and following principles of a low-carbohydrate diet (even if they're not on a diet!). As a result, these patients fear certain foods such as bread, pasta and grains, because they have been led to believe that eating carbs is the reason they are overweight. Many of them are also under the impression that certain fruits are 'fattening' because they have read or been told that they have a high sugar content.

Of course, all of this is nonsense – it couldn't be further from the truth – but it takes time for people to trust and understand how the body reacts to certain food intake. Unlearning everything you think you know about food and exercise certainly is a challenge!

As a result of following some sort of low-carb diet, patients are then quick to complain, when first starting the IWL plan, that their weight has gone up since eating carbs again. Carbs have been a common scapegoat for all our weight problems for decades. Carbs are made up of many sugar units bundled together to form glycogen. As it turns out, each gram of carbohydrate binds three grams of water. So, as you can imagine, this ends up weighing quite a bit. But it's no reason for concern, because all you're experiencing when you add carbs back to your daily eating plan is an increase in water content in your body.

If you're one of those people (don't worry, many of us are) who have been on some form of low-carb eating plan and then introduce the principles of the IWL plan into your everyday life, the number on the scales is likely to go up. But, I strongly emphasise that this is not an increase in true weight or fat mass but rather an increase in water content in the body. In fact, carbs (the healthy type, not the sugar-coated processed stuff) are going to help you lose the weight and will become one of the key weapons in your weight-loss arsenal. Be excited by this – you can eat carbs and lose weight as a result!

It's important to include plenty of wholegrain carbohydrate sources as part of the IWL plan. These foods are packed with nutrients and high in fibre. These are also the foods that are going to help prevent diseases such as type 2 diabetes and heart disease.

As they are high in fibre, it is important to gradually introduce them into your diet to prevent stomach upsets such as gas and bloating. If you find you can't tolerate bread, try a variety from your local baker, or eliminate bread from your diet. You don't have to eat bread, but you do have to include wholegrain carbs. There are plenty of great wholegrain carbs you can include in your IWL plan (I'll explain these in Chapter 8). However, as I explain later, and particularly relevant during pregnancy, bread is also fortified with iodine and folate – two key nutrients that are needed for the healthy development of a baby if you are pregnant.

So, if you have been following a low-carb diet and then have suddenly switched to the IWL plan, don't be disheartened when you see the number on the scales go up with the reintroduction of healthy wholegrain carbohydrates. It's just water and will correct over time. By including a wash-out period of at least one month to ensure your weight stabilises, you will come to terms with this adjustment and not jump to the wrong conclusion.

Previous diets

The next thing to consider is if you are currently following any form of diet. In this instance, you must get off it immediately to prevent further harm to your body. Think back to the biological protections that I explained in the first chapter. If you have recently finished a diet and have not yet regained all the weight you lost, you will most likely have to wait until your body fights back to its set point. I'm not going to sugar-coat it: your body is likely in lockdown, depending on how much weight you lost and how drastic a measure you took. But the good news is you can speed up the process by implementing all the principles of the IWL plan, which may result in your weight stabilising earlier. This will allow your body to recover from the stress and, importantly, reverse the damage you have inflicted on it from dieting. Don't expect to see weight loss from the outset, but do expect to see psychological improvements and an increased quality of life after you start implementing the IWL plan.

Flashback to Melissa, whom I introduced at the start of the chapter. Melissa completed her homework over the four weeks. She read the *Interval Weight Loss For Life* book and tracked her weight each week. She felt dismayed by her progress as the number escalated on the scales the entire time. She was already willing to give up. In fact, by the time I saw her four weeks later, she had regained all the weight she lost on the keto diet. Her husband, Pete, was very supportive and had also read the book several times to ensure he could support her every step of the way. He had come to the realisation that he too had a weight problem, and that it was not to be ruled out when it came to the real problem at hand – a failure to conceive. In fact, up to 30 per cent of infertility problems can be attributed to the male.

Melissa was convinced this was the heaviest weight she had been at her entire life, but just to make sure her weight was not still rebounding from the recent stresses she had imposed on her body, I convinced her that she should have another wash-out month. She was feeling much more energetic and happier now that she could enjoy carbs again, but she still saw them as the cause of her problem due to the increase in weight they had introduced to the scales. After much convincing (mainly from Pete), Melissa took another wash-out month following the IWL plan. She continued to track her weight once a week and was not to focus on weight loss. Pete also began the journey as he needed to do something about his weight and support her along the way.

Are there exceptions to the wash-out rule?

There are exceptions. If you are confident that you are currently at your set point and don't have a history of dieting, you will see success on the IWL plan from the get-go. But if you've been a serial dieter, it's no need for concern. The wash-out month gives you ample time to wrap your head around the six principles of the plan and how to apply it to your lifestyle. Importantly, it will still work for you but you need to shift your mindset from the quick-fix mentality. Remember, this is not a program that will see you skinny in a couple of months' time only to have you stack it back on just as quickly. Instead, the IWL plan will see you progressively lighter and healthier for the rest of your life, with never a thought of diets or worrying about your weight again. You can't change the past, but you can change your future.

General rule of thumb

Even if you have recently been on a diet and regained all the weight you lost, it doesn't hurt to implement a wash-out month on the IWL plan, just to make sure you have all your ducks in a row before initiating a weight-loss month. You also need to make sure your weight is stable. I cannot repeat this enough: you must ensure your weight has stabilised before starting out on a weight-loss month.

Two months after first meeting Melissa, she was now confident that she was at her set point. This was 92 kilograms, 32 kilograms more than her lightest weight as an adult; a far cry from the 60 kilograms she reported weighing in her youth. She was very sad at the thought of this and reported how she had spent thousands of dollars on various diets, online programs, pills and shakes over the years. But the great news was that her weight had stabilised over the second month of her wash-out period; it increased the first month, and then continued to increase during the second month from weeks 4 to 6 (91–92.4 kilograms) but then stabilised from weeks 6 to 8 (92.4–92 kilograms). Her husband, Pete, had also monitored his weight during the second month of Melissa's wash-out and it was stable, ranging from 95.6 kilograms to 95.8 kilograms, which meant he was at his set point. He was also confident that this was the heaviest he had ever been, based on his clothes size and not dieting in the past. Melissa was very excited and ready to start a weight-loss month of the IWL plan. But, before she did, we needed to calculate her, and her husband's, new goal set point; a realistic weight loss they could both achieve and maintain.

The definition of a healthy body weight

Social media, reality TV shows and magazines have created a very unhealthy portrayal of a healthy body weight. Those images of people at home wearing full TV make-up, being snapped by a professional photographer and edited by an app that pinches in their waist are fantasies. These people don't actually look anything like that in real life. Everyone's body shape is different, and it is not helpful to set out to look like those you follow on social media. In fact, it can be downright dangerous, and if you have a habit of doing so, perhaps this can be one of the goals you need to address while following the IWL plan – that is, to stop scrolling through social media. Whatever amount of weight you want to lose, do not compare yourself to other people, because that is neither healthy nor realistic. Focus on your individual goals and a sustainable weight-loss plan for yourself.

What other indicators can you use?

Aside from body weight, waist circumference is just as valuable a tool for monitoring your change over time. Waist circumference complements your body weight measure for a better picture of your risk of metabolic disease. Your health is at risk if your waist size is greater than 80 cm (about 31.5 inches) for women, and for the men reading this, greater than 94 cm (about 37 inches). However, guidelines vary for different ethnicities. There are different guidelines for people from Asia, and those from South and Central America, with a recommended cut-off of 80 cm for women and 90 cm for men. This does not apply during pregnancy. I stress that you should not worry about your weight gain or waist circumference increase during pregnancy.

It is best to get someone to assist you when completing a waist circumference measure for best accuracy. You can simply place the tape around the point of your belly button and you should do it on bare skin for consistency. There is a useful online calculator at the government website Health Direct to help you assess the health risk of your current waist circumference and body mass index (BMI) – another somewhat useful tool.

BMI is used in a clinical setting to calculate whether a person is in a healthy body weight range. It is calculated as your weight over your height squared. So, for someone who is 180 cm tall and weighs 100 kg, their BMI is 30.9 kg/m^2 (calculated as $100/(1.8 \times 1.8) = 100/3.24 = 30.86$. For men and women, a healthy BMI is between 18.5 and 24.9 kg/m^2. However, the major limitation with this tool is that it doesn't take into consideration a person's muscle mass so it's a complete waste of time for athletes. The cut-off points were also derived predominantly from data from North American and European populations and are not applicable to all ethnic groups. This issue has led to suggested redefined BMI cut-off points for people of Asian ethnicity (where a BMI of more than 23.0 is defined as overweight, and more than 27.5 as obese) and for those of Polynesian ethnicity, with a BMI cut-off point of more than 26 for overweight and more than 32 for obese.

Don't worry if this all seems a bit complicated. Just jump on the government website Health Direct to see whether yours sits within a healthy range: www.healthdirect.gov.au/bmi-calculator. However, you will need someone to measure your height and you may need to get your doctor to do this.

When it comes to problems with weight, we all like to blame our genes. But the truth is, genetics are not to blame for the increasing prevalence of obesity; our genes haven't changed over time and we still have the same genes as our ancestors. Our DNA contains all our different genes – hundreds of thousands of them. But 98 per cent of our DNA's function remains a mystery. Therefore, as you can guess, mutations in a segment of DNA that regulates gene expression – the ones that enable life – are very rare and affect around 2 per cent of the population. Many of us have a genetic predisposition to obesity but it has no consequence because our genetic make-up is just a predisposition, not an inevitable fate. This means you can lose weight just as effectively as the person next to you, irrespective of your genetic make-up. This is good news for you and will save you all those thousands of dollars that you may have contemplated on DNA testing; it is a waste of time and money, and just another identity-excuse that we search for. It doesn't matter if you need to lose 10 kilograms, 20 kilograms or more than 50 kilograms – anyone can follow and succeed on the IWL plan, but there are certain things to take into consideration when determining your weight-loss goal. Defining a realistic and achievable new 'set point' is the first step towards success on the IWL plan.

Your tasks

Step 1

Write down your set point – both weight and waist circumference – on the top of a large palm card. This is your current body weight after following the steps in this chapter to ensure you are at your set point. Everyone's is different, so don't compare with your friend.

Let's flash back to Melissa and her husband, Pete. Melissa's body weight after the two-month wash-out period stabilised at 92 kilograms. Her body weight was 60 kilograms seventeen years ago but is now 92 kilograms, the heaviest weight she has been. In this case, her set point is not 60 kilograms but 92 kilograms (her current weight after the wash-out period on the IWL plan). This is the weight (92 kilograms) that Melissa wrote down on the top of her palm card.

Step 2

Now I want you to write down on the same palm card, on the bottom section, the lowest body weight you have been in your adult years. If you're not entirely sure, put down what you think it was. For Melissa this was 60 kilograms at age eighteen, before she went to university.

Step 3

Lastly, you are going to write down your goal set point in big numbers in the middle section of the palm card. Let's flash back to Melissa and Pete again to help you with this process.

Melissa's goal was not to achieve her previous lowest weight of 60 kilograms. This was most likely unrealistic, and also unnecessary for her health. Instead, we chose a new set point that was between her lowest weight as an adult and her current set point. The perfect starting point for Melissa was 76 kilograms, or a weight loss of approximately 16 kilograms. We know that losing just 3 kilograms can lead to significant improvements in health markers like cholesterol, and can also reduce your chances of dying from cardiovascular disease. Melissa wanted to fall pregnant again, so this could potentially happen at any stage beyond a 3 kilogram weight loss, but until it did, she would continue losing weight.

Her husband, Pete, was at his highest ever body weight – 95.8 kilograms – and he recorded this on his own palm card. He was now thirty-eight and recalled his lowest body weight being 80 kilograms when he was playing rugby at university. For Pete we set a new goal set point of 85 kilograms. This equated to an 11 kilogram weight loss.

Melissa wrote down 76 kilograms in the middle of her card and Pete recorded 85 kilograms.

For you, this palm card will be your reference point and should be placed in a highly visible spot where you can always see it. Everyone needs to start with a realistic goal and then reassess this goal *after* they achieve it. A good starting point for your goal set point is the mid-point between your lowest body weight and your current weight. You won't get there any slower by doing this – this is the IWL way (I'll explain in the next chapter).

Don't worry if this all seems a little much, because you can also get your very own personalised weight tracker using the IWL online program, available through the Interval Weight Loss website.

CHAPTER 6

THE FIRST PRINCIPLE:
YOU CAN'T FIGHT EVOLUTION

You now know why you haven't succeeded on your weight-loss journey to date. Just as the problem is evolutionary, so too is the solution. Which brings me to explain the very first principle of the IWL plan: *You can't fight evolution.* Recall your set point – the weight at which your body is most comfortable and the weight that you are most likely at now. This is the underlying foundation of why the IWL plan works; it allows you to redefine your set point by following a plan that prevents your body's usual response to weight loss, to ensure that the strong biological drivers that have prevented you from succeeding in the past stay dormant and don't come into play. Every second month you will be required to maintain the weight loss from the month before to allow your body to recalibrate the set point. This helps your body to get used to the new set point before it can move on to further weight loss.

Your goal weight loss per month

When you impose a stress on your body (as with dieting), it starts to work differently and will slow down to counteract the weight loss. Losing only 2–3 kilograms – the weight loss we consider clinically significant – can trigger this process in the body. The reason this weight loss is considered significant in a clinical setting is because, if sustained, it will result in an improvement in metabolic health and reduce your chance of dying prematurely from heart disease.

Bearing this in mind, with the IWL plan, the general rule of thumb is to stick to a 2 kilogram weight loss over the course of a month (approximately 0.5 kilogram weight loss per week) to safely ensure that you prevent the usual biological responses kicking into gear. It is then crucial to maintain that 2 kilogram weight loss for the second month (i.e. stay at the same weight for the second month) before going on to lose weight again during the third month, and so on, until your goal weight loss is achieved.

To help you better understand the application of the first principle of the IWL plan – *You can't fight evolution* – I want you to visualise a hunter–gatherer or cave dweller. Your role is to stop the cave dweller getting upset, but this will only happen if you stick to the 2 kilogram weight-loss goal and allow the dweller to rest every other month.

If you continue to lose weight during the weight-maintenance months, the IWL plan becomes just another stress on your body and you will get the same response that you have had every other time: your body will go into protection mode and you will go back to where you started. All the biological protections that you learnt about in the first chapter – metabolism, appetite hormones, energy sources, thyroid and adrenal gland function, and brain function – will kick into gear unless you allow your body to rest. The same applies if you lose more than the clinically significant amount of weight per month (more than 2 kilograms) – you will also fail because the same innate physiological responses will kick in.

This generally means no more than a 12 kilogram weight loss over the course of a year. I know! Many of you are probably rolling your eyes thinking, *Gosh, this is going to be a long journey.* Yes, it's going to seem longer initially but it's going to seem fast when your friend who lost the 10 kilograms of water, muscle and fat in four weeks on the latest diet is trying to play catch-up when they stack it back on.

Everyone knows somebody – most likely multiple some-bodies – who has done the latest and greatest diet, only to end up a size bigger than they originally were. The IWL plan requires patience and will challenge those who are looking for instant results. Even though you won't lose the weight as quickly as you're used to, you're going to be much better off. And if you take the fixation off weight loss and instead place the focus on forming new habits, the weight will naturally drop. There will be no more staring longingly at a piece of chocolate because you've cut out sugar only to binge on McDonald's on the way home, and there will be no more hating how you feel when you fail – because you will. Everyone is familiar with the tortoise-and-hare parable – slow and steady wins the race. Trust me, your friends will only be looking for the next diet that hits the shelves in a desperate attempt to catch up to you at six or 12 months.

How to track your weight

A key part of your success on the IWL plan relates to tracking your body weight so that you can make the small but often necessary adjustments to achieve your goal set point. It's important, therefore, to have access to a reliable set of scales. You can track your weight using the Interval Weight Loss online program or by using an electronic spreadsheet (an example is available for free download at intervalweightloss.com.au). You must record your weight data so you can visually analyse the trend over time. An increase or decrease of a couple of hundred grams on the scales does not mean your weight has changed. However, if your weight was going down a couple of hundred grams every week over the course of the month, this would be indicative of weight loss, because the trend is going down.

It's a waste of time to simply weigh yourself and say you will remember the weight next week when you weigh in, because all too often we forget. It is also a waste of time just writing your weight down on a piece of paper each week, unless it is visually plotted on a graph. By observing the trend over time – week by week – you can determine whether you are losing weight and dropping fat (you will drop fat and hold onto your muscle if you follow the steps outlined in this book). Remember, you shouldn't be losing too much weight or continuing to lose weight during the weight-maintenance months.

How often should you track it?

You need to commit to weighing yourself weekly. Focusing on every little change in your body weight from meal to meal and from day to day is not what you should be doing, because body weight fluctuates enormously over the course of a day, and weighing too often will be misleading. For many of us, this is a common scenario – we jump on the scales repeatedly throughout the day and worry about every little ounce of weight change. We think that an increase of 500 grams after a high-carb meal is true weight change, which leads me to a very interesting and fun project I encourage you to try. Weigh yourself 10 times over the course of the day and see for yourself how much your weight fluctuates.

Sorry to put a dampener on your experiment, but your weight can fluctuate by as much as 1–2 kilograms in any given day depending on your current weight, what stage of your menstrual cycle you are at, what you have eaten, how much fluid you have drunk and how much exercise you have done. These day-to-day fluctuations are completely normal and largely due to the amount of water in your body; they are not a change in fat mass. Do not be concerned by them.

When should you weigh yourself?

I want you to jump on the same scales at the same time and day each week. For consistency, weigh yourself in your underwear first thing before breakfast. It is important to use the same set of scales, because there can be a huge discrepancy between different scales. If you are unsure of which brand of scales to buy, go to your local sports store and talk to the staff to determine your best value for money. Choose scales with a large electronic display that makes it easy to read the weight, and be sure to change the batteries regularly. A body-weight recording is the only thing you need. Many of the scales will provide all sorts of data including body-fat analyses, but these are largely misleading and inaccurate and you shouldn't take note of these values.

The only exception to weekly weighing is during pregnancy. This is a time when you don't need to track your weight. Weight gain is healthy and expected, and the last thing you need to worry about is how much you are putting on, providing you are following the other principles of the IWL plan (with the increased food allowance to cater for the baby you are growing). More detail is provided on this later in the chapter.

What should your weight-loss trend look like?

When observing your body weight, the key is to analyse the trend over time. If your weight goes from 82.2 kilograms in week 1, to 82.0 in week 2, to 82.5 in week 3, and then 82.4 in week 4, this would be considered weight maintenance and not weight gain. In this example, the decrease from week 1 to week 2 is also unlikely to be weight loss, unless the trend continued to decrease in following weeks. For example, from 82.2 kilograms in week 1, to 82.0 in week 2, to 81.9 in week 3, to 81.7 in week 4.

Don't read too much into one measurement on the scales, because it doesn't provide anything meaningful. If you are in the middle of a weight-loss period, the trend should be going down 1–2 kilograms over the month, and if it is a weight-maintenance month it should be stable across the month in order to reset your body weight. You will never have a perfect weight trajectory – it is just the trend you are looking for. Some months you might only lose 0.5 kilograms, but this is still success. This is also especially relevant to those who wish to lose just a few kilograms. For example, if you have set a 5 kilogram weight-loss goal, it is more realistic to aim for a 0.5–1 kilogram weight loss per month, rather than 2 kilograms.

Importantly, the task of tracking your body weight will teach you how it responds to different stimuli. Later chapters teach you how to adjust your lifestyle in accordance with what your weight trajectory is doing; that is, methods and tips you can use if you are failing to achieve weight loss or if you are struggling to maintain your weight during a weight-maintenance month. This is also made available through the IWL personalised weight tracker as part of the online program. The structured weekly plans will provide you with examples of what to do each month to ensure you optimise your success. An example recording chart for a patient for both a weight-loss period and a weight-maintenance period are as follows.

(A) Body-weight tracker for weight-loss month

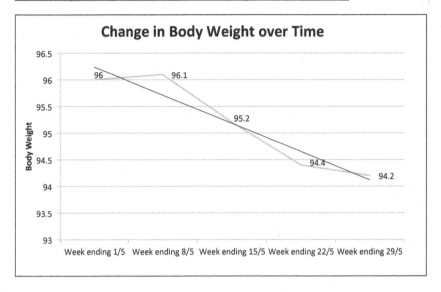

The key thing to look for on this graph is the trend over time – that is, it is going down over the course of the month (approximate 2 kilogram weight loss from starting point – day 0 – of 96.0 kilograms). The straight black line is the linear trend, which is what you want to observe over time. It is also important to ensure you are not losing more than 0.5 kilograms per week. If you see it going down by more than 0.5 kilograms per week, you need to ease off and adjust your IWL plan, as outlined in Chapters 12 and 14. No weight-loss trajectory is ever picture perfect. Don't panic if the weight loss varies from week to week – this is normal. For example, a weight change from 96.0 to 96.3 kilograms is not weight gain unless the following week you witness it go up again to, say, 96.8 kilograms. If you see the trend going down over the month, then you are perfectly on track!

(B) Body-weight tracker for weight-maintenance month

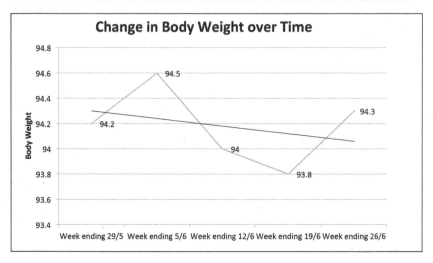

As with the previous example, the key thing to observe in this graph is the trend over time. Note the trend evens out over the course of the month to maintain the 2 kilogram weight loss from the previous month. This is extremely important, because continued weight loss will result in failure. The black line is the linear trend. In this graph, the variations in body weight are considered weight maintenance. Your weight should stay within 1 kilogram either side of your previous month's weight loss over the entire weight-maintenance month.

(C) Body-weight tracker for weight-maintenance month

This is an example where there is a trend towards weight loss over the first two weeks (from 94.2 kilograms at the end of a weight-loss period in Graph (A) to 93.5 kilograms on week ending 5/6 and 93.4 kilograms on week ending 12/6). However, because this is in a weight-maintenance month, the person has corrected this by adjusting their IWL plan to ensure their body weight corrects back to the starting point of the weight-maintenance month (which was 94.2 kilograms). In Chapter 14 I will elaborate further on how you

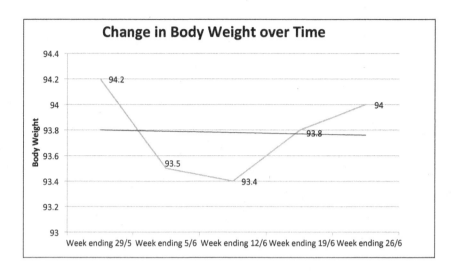

can make these compensatory changes. A weight trajectory from 94.2 to 94.0 kilograms over the month is considered weight maintenance and definitely not weight loss. If this person's weight was 94.5 kilograms at the end of the weight-maintenance period, this would also be considered success. In fact, it is success even if you keep within 1 kilogram either side of your previous month, but it is much safer to be within 0.5 kilograms.

(D) Body-weight tracker for 12-month period

Note that in this 12-month chart the weight is decreasing by approximately 2 kilograms each month and then maintained for the following month, equating to approximately a 12 kilogram weight loss over an entire year. The weight loss is not perfect and never will be. Your goal is to simply monitor the trend in change over time. Body weight is 96.3 kilograms at baseline and 84.4 kilograms after approximately 12 months. You can see that some months have resulted in very little weight loss and others a little more. The most important thing is that small amounts of weight loss are followed by months of weight maintenance.

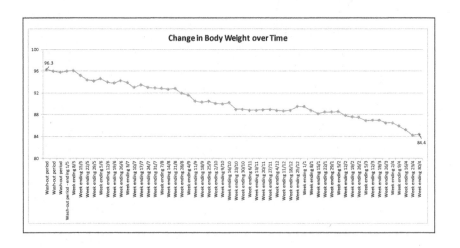

Your task

First, you need to get some scales. Your next step is to download the Interval Weight Loss online program to enable you to track your weight with feedback as you progress. There is also a recording template you can download from the Interval Weight Loss website. Leave this weight tracker with your scales so that you can record your weight every week on the same day and at the same time.

Start today and weigh yourself every single week. This will help you develop an understanding of how your body works so that you can begin to make small modifications over time.

CHAPTER 7

THE SECOND PRINCIPLE:
REACH FOR NATURE FIRST

Just like the first principle of the IWL plan, the second principle requires us to take a deeper look at our ancestors. Recall that during our time as hunter–gatherers food was hard to come by and often calories were scarce. We therefore learnt to seek out foods that were high in energy and that were palatable. This was needed in order to survive. During our ancestors' time these were foods that were found in nature – foods that were high in sugar, such as fruits and honey, and foods that were high in fat such as meat and nuts. It is no shock that these foods also gave us pleasure. They would release those feel-good chemicals in the brain every time we ate them, which subsequently shaped our food choices. Fast-forward a few hundred thousand years to the modern-day environment and now the story is different. Of course, our instinct is to still search for pleasure-seeking foods, but now we get those highs from fast food, confectionary and soft drinks. A far cry from nature's treats that we once sought.

Just as we haven't evolved from the evolutionary propensity to protect against weight loss (the first principle of the IWL plan – *You can't fight evolution*), we also haven't evolved from ancient survival circuits in the brain (the second principle of the IWL plan – *Reach for nature first*). As mentioned earlier in the book, this is known as an evolutionary mismatch, meaning that evolved traits that were once advantageous become harmful when placed in a foreign environment. In the case of food, our calorie-seeking brains were a useful trait when food was hard to come by, but unfortunately this is not the case when submerged in the modern-day environment saturated with food. We simply can't control ourselves. Learning how to retrain the brain to *reach for nature first* is a very important component of the IWL plan and the second of six key principles to success.

Nature's treats

Food that gives us pleasure is tasty and therefore hard to resist. Much like the high we get from having sex or listening to great music, we find that satisfaction from food (specifically those foods that are high in fat or sugar).

When we register a pleasure, endorphins are released simultaneously with dopamine into the brain's pleasure centre called the nucleus accumbens. The brain then remembers this sense of satisfaction and triggers a response the next time we see the food. However, the pleasure once derived from fruits, vegetables, honey, nuts and seeds – nature's treats – has been hijacked. Instead of being 'wired' to rely on foods in their natural state, we have become 'wired' to rely on heavily processed manufactured foods. These foods are low in nutrition and very high in calories; they cause cravings when we see them, and they can result in overconsumption due to a loss of control when eating them. The added fat, salt and sugars in these foods trigger addictive-like eating behaviours, which we see in our modern obsession with so many foods such as cakes, chips, pastries, chocolates, pizza and hamburgers.

The 'wiring' of the brain

The human brain contains neurons – approximately 100 billion of them. Each neuron in the brain has a long cable – several times thinner than a human hair – called an axon, and this is where signals from the neuron travel away to be received by other neurons. These neurons have synaptic connections (up to 100,000) formed from other neurons, that allow them to communicate to one another. This is effectively referred to as the 'wiring' in the brain.

The good news is the 'hardwiring' of the brain is in fact 'soft-wiring' that can be retrained. What I am telling you is that you can change the wiring of your brain and it does respond to new situations, environments and lifestyles. However, this is not easy and the first few months on the IWL plan are the most challenging. A lifetime of poor food choices based on fast food may mean it requires a little more persistence. But eventually you will become less reliant on those foods through consistent and positive food choices.

Forming new habits

Your brain is made up of both grey and white matter. In order to better understand how the brain works when it comes to food choices, we must look at an area called the prefrontal cortex. This section of the brain is made up of grey matter (containing plenty of those neurons I just described) and is the part of the brain that makes decisions – the lifestyle choices you make. Unhealthy lifestyle choices (for example, reaching for the daily croissant or can of Coke) can lead to a change in the structure of the pre-frontal cortex and an unfavourable decline in the volume of grey matter in the brain. However, the opposite also applies, in that you can increase the grey matter volume and connectivity of neurons in the prefrontal cortex by repeatedly applying positive meal choices. This will mean healthier food choices then become easier as time goes on. The best way to think of your brain is to consider how a muscle responds to training. If you train it repeatedly, it will strengthen over time. And a major step to adapting to success is making that very first positive choice. Repeatedly applying correct choices will see you re-wiring your brain over time and, consequently, result in success.

This ability to say *no* is not just limited to the instances when we are alone. The same can be said of our support networks – our friends, family and colleagues. Your ability to stick to your goals is highly influenced by others. For example, there is some cheese and wine on the table and your girlfriends are having a good time. How do you say *no* to a drink or the cheese when you would previously always say *yes*? As a tribal society, people are made uncomfortable by those breaking the mould. Even though your decision to decline that drink and cheese will be difficult, because you are breaking from that tribal mould, it is the choice that you need to make. But this doesn't mean saying *no* all the time. That is certainly not the IWL way!

The IWL plan doesn't impose any bans on foods. We can all cut certain foods for a period – typically one to three months – but cravings for high-fat and high-sugar foods will come back with a vengeance. Recall from the first chapter that research utilising brain imaging has confirmed this – there is a heightened activity of the limbic (reward) system in the brain following weight loss, which drives an increased desire for those foods that have been cut from the diet. This is exactly why the IWL plan doesn't take this approach – having access to those favourite bad foods will ensure you succeed with your long-term weight-loss goals.

Sustainable success

When you give something up you always feel its loss. Giving up what we love makes us feel resentful and angry, and that we are missing out. Eventually, in the psychology of missing out we say something along the lines of, 'Stuff it, I'm going to do what I want,' which normally means a return to the bad habit. This is the classic Yin and Yang of internal dialogue, another way of describing the angel and the devil within us, which guides our every reaction.

So, with the wine and cheese example just mentioned, while it requires you to consistently promote self-control, it doesn't require you to cut it out completely. The same can be said with the McDonald's drive-through, the bag of crisps from the vending machine or the piece of chocolate that your colleague offers you at work; it doesn't mean you can never have it, but it does mean you need to be able to say *no* most of the time. In the modern environment we are presented with these choices all the time. They have become more than the occasional appearance at a birthday or celebration; they have become part of our daily ritual. Developing the ability to say *no* and gain control over your food choices is vital to success on the IWL plan.

How long will it take?

Many people have unrealistic expectations about the speed, ease and consequences of changing a behaviour. Irrespective of what you are trying to achieve, actual change takes time, effort and patience. However, this is not always a linear process and it is normal to take a backward step at times. Research has proven that it takes 66 days to create a new habit or to break an old one. Yes, that's right, it takes more than two months before a new behaviour becomes automatic and you can beat the addiction.

After you break through this 66-day barrier, you will notice an improvement in your behaviour and ease in being able to restrain or implement self-control when it comes to food choices. You will gain the ability to restrain or exercise self-control over what you eat. The first 66 days are the hardest, but I promise you'll be reaching for the mangoes and salmon soon!

How to beat the addiction

1. If you are currently eating your favourite nutrient-poor foods every day – it could be the croissant, the banana bread, the chocolate bar, the can of Coke or the McDonald's drive-through – the goal is to reduce the frequency of these foods gradually. Using a diary, write down every time you have a treat food. Count these up each week and slowly work towards an intake of one treat per week on the weight-loss months of the IWL plan and to two per week on the weight-maintenance months (more on this later). It may take longer to achieve your goal with this weaning process but it's an effective approach, and like all things IWL, it rewards those who play the long game.

2. Find some naturally occurring foods high in sugar and fat that you love and surround yourself with them. Every time you feel that urge to eat something sugary or fatty coming on, *reach for nature first* – fruits, honey, nuts, seeds and avocado are a few suitable examples. It really doesn't matter what you have, if you *reach for nature first*. You will get the same high you usually get from all the processed sweets and fatty foods because nature's treats also light up our brain's dopamine receptors and release those feel-good chemicals. If you stick to this, the cravings for the junk food will eventually fade. Be prepared, though, to ride out that 66-day barrier to break the habit. It's worth it. Strawberries, berries, watermelon, mangoes, pink lady apples, nuts, seeds, and honey or avocado on wholegrain toast all make great snacks.

3. Buy single-serve packages of chocolate, ice-cream, biscuits, chips or whatever your favourite treats might be. This enforces the portion size you can have without the risk

of you devouring the entire packet. Make sure it's something you really love – you want to make it a worthwhile treat and you want to savour every bite.

4. Keep the treats out of sight so you don't see them every time you open the fridge or cupboard. Always keep healthy foods visible and at eye level. On the front of your fridge place the six principles of the IWL plan to remind yourself at all times to *reach for nature first*.

5. Every time you get a sugar craving, try taking just a taste. By allowing yourself a few bites you get maximum enjoyment for minimal damage. Research has proven this – the first bite of any treat food yields the most pleasure. A great way to implement this is by challenging yourself to see how long you can keep just one piece of chocolate in your mouth.

6. Cut down on impulse eating by delaying pleasure. For example, tell yourself you can have the McDonald's burger, pizza, chocolate bar or ice-cream after you complete that task on your 'to do' list (you will learn about this shortly); you make it harder to access the treat, but you are not saying no. Once we get absorbed in a task, we often forget all about the craving because we're so happy to have finished the job and want to continue a good streak.

7. Consider whether you are hungry or just bored. Reach for a glass of water or herbal tea and remove yourself from technology. If you are still feeling hungry after following these steps, *reach for nature first*.

8. Record your expenditure. A simple task that involves recording all your food intake can often prompt you to eat out less often and to buy fewer treats and takeaway meals. My wife and I do this all the time to keep track of where we could be

better saving. Buying food on-the-go or convenience foods all the time can be very expensive. The most effective way of becoming aware of how much you can save is by recording your daily food cost. You can usually get four home-cooked meals for the price of one dining-out meal, which will have a huge effect on your bank balance over time and make you more aware of your food choices.

Your tasks

Task 1

Starting today, you need to start saying *no* to the office cake and sweets, the afternoon wine and cheese, and the banana bread at the cafe with your friend. Save these treats for special occasions – once per week on the weight-loss months and twice per week on the weight-maintenance months. You need to record in your diary or on your phone each time you have one and tally them up each week so that you can reduce the frequency of them over time. Remember, I'm not telling you to exclude them altogether – you can still include them in your weekly treat count (more on this to come in later chapters).

Task 2

Start recording how much you spend each day on food. Sit down with your partner or a friend, or alone if you prefer, and tally it up at the end of each week. This is a fun task to see how much you can save by simply preparing more food at home. It's also a great excuse to regularly catch up with friends or family to share your progress.

CHAPTER 8

THE THIRD PRINCIPLE: FULL RAINBOW

Food is the life source we need to nourish the body and help it get back to its natural preferred weight – its *set point*. Food is your ally and your body will thrive if you give it the right fuel. It needs nutritious and wholesome food. For decades we have been taught that weight loss is all about restricting our food intake. Restriction and dieting have become a cultural obsession, but this is the very last thing you should be doing when embarking on your weight-loss journey, as the body learns to store food and fat when food is restricted. Instead, the focus needs to be on having more nutritious and wholesome food and an abundance of variety; eating more, not less!

When you embrace wholesome, nutritious foods (see the list of foods later in this chapter) you will lose the fear of food that you have had for so long and it will become something you enjoy and that fuels your life, rather than something that controls you. You will lose the belief that the more you eat the fatter you will become, as so many of my patients have assumed, and you will also see the number on the scales go down. Inadvertently, the increase in food and change in foods you are eating will result in a reduction in your calorie intake. Restricting your food intake will only result in your body's functioning slowing down and you won't get the weight-loss results you are after. There are no foods that you need to exclude when following the IWL plan, and every time you sit down to a meal the plate should include each of the three macro-nutrients (fat, wholegrain carbohydrate and protein) and different colours to ensure you get in your daily quota of salad and vegetables. This is the third principle of the IWL plan – *Full rainbow*.

The IWL plan brings back the pleasure to eating food that so many lose when they obsessively diet, meaning people find it an easy and sustainable approach to changing their lifestyle.

In many instances, people don't start to lose weight on the IWL plan until they increase their food intake. It seems ridiculous, I know, but remember that the body has learnt to defend itself during times of starvation – it will slow down during times of restriction and speed up during times of abundance.

What foods should you eat on the IWL plan?

Simple, whole foods are the most satisfying and therefore these are the foods that you need to include in abundance on the IWL plan. When foods are tested in the laboratory, they give us a value that scientists refer to as the satiety index. Foods that are low in satiety and not as filling include refined sources such as white bread, cake, croissants and other bakery goods. On the other hand, foods that are high on the satiety index and that fill you up for long periods of time include fruit, potatoes, beans and meat. They are foods found in their natural state and typically high in fibre and protein. Bearing this in mind, the basis of your daily food intake on the IWL plan should include the following.

1. Unlimited fruit and vegetables (all are suitable, but enjoy a variety). I don't care what anyone tells you, you can never eat too many fruits and vegetables.

2. Plenty (two to three serves per day) of dairy products (milk and yoghurt) or suitable dairy-free alternative foods (more on what they do later in this chapter).

3. Cheese only once per week.

4. A handful of nuts and seeds.

5. Inclusion of a wholegrain carbohydrate with three meals per day. For example, wholegrain bread, wholegrain pasta, brown rice, barley, buckwheat, oats, quinoa.

6. Plenty of fish or seafood with at least three meals per week.

7. Inclusion of protein – lean or 'heart smart' cuts of meat (trim all visible forms of fat off the meat), tofu, legumes (all types) or eggs with each of the three main meals per day. (It is important to note that not every meal needs to be meat – plant-based meals are an important part of the IWL plan.)

8. Treats (i.e. ice-cream, chocolate, biscuits, burgers, pizzas, bakery food) no more than once per week in the weight-loss months and twice per week in the weight-maintenance months.

9. Fast food or dining out no more than once per week in the weight-loss months and twice per week in the weight-maintenance months.

10. A glass of water before every meal and at times when you think you are hungry.

What foods should you avoid during pregnancy?

There is no need to become fixated on what you should and shouldn't eat during pregnancy, but there are a couple of high-risk foods that you should avoid, reducing risk to you and your baby. This is because some foods pose a higher risk of containing harmful bacteria, such as listeria and salmonella, and it's mainly applicable when the foods are raw. Foods to avoid include raw eggs, raw seafood, soft cheeses, raw meat, ready-to-eat luncheon meats (for example, deli meats), pate, sushi, pre-prepared or packaged salads, fruit and sandwiches (including salad bars and smorgasbords) and raw beansprouts. Anything ready-to-eat is best avoided. You can still enjoy a range of foods, but you need to cook them. Cooking food at risk of contamination kills off the bacteria and makes it safe to eat (for example, eggs, soft cheese, fish and meat), or you need to prepare the foods from scratch yourself, for example, sushi, salads and sandwiches. And you can still have cheese! But it needs to be hard cheese such as cheddar, instead of soft cheeses such as brie, camembert, ricotta or feta. There is a great infographic on foods best to avoid available at the Health Direct website: pregnancybirthbaby.org.au/guide-to-food-and-drink-during-pregnancy.

Quantity of food during pregnancy

The same principle that applies for everyone following the IWL plan applies during pregnancy. You should be focusing on including plenty of food, listening and responding to your hunger cues and never depriving yourself of nutrition. During the first two trimesters you may not notice much change in your appetite, however this will change during the third trimester (from week 28 onwards) when your baby grows quickly and lays down stores of fat. This is a time when you may need one and a third times the quantity of food that is prescribed on the IWL plan (I will give you an indication of portion sizes to get your started later in the book).

Grocery shopping

Grocery shopping is not easy. Supermarkets are designed to guide us around the perimeter of the store and to make trips up and down the aisles. Unsurprisingly, therefore, products located at the end of the aisles and checkout-counter displays account for nearly half of all sales. They are stacked with soft drinks, sweets, chips and bakery goods.

To limit your exposure to these foods, your grocery shopping should be done once a week. If you really don't trust yourself in the supermarket or if you find yourself eating a chocolate bar or packet of chips every time you go there, you should consider ordering everything online and having it delivered. It is much better to do that than succumb to those impulse buys and poor food choices when at the supermarket. For those with children it can also be a less stressful experience as you avoid facing the risk of your kid having a tantrum or having them nagging you the whole time to buy junk. In addition, the extra time you've saved from that risky shopping expedition can be devoted to some structured physical activity or one of your hobbies. The weekly food shop will not change much from week to week, which makes ordering online even easier as your foods will be saved from the previous week's purchase.

If you are going to hit the shops, it's important to take a list with you to ensure you don't forget anything (I provide you with one in this chapter), because that will only result in your having to go back to the supermarket mid-week. Not only will it reduce your chance of succumbing to temptation, it can save you money. It's also vital to have a contingency plan in case your kid does throw a tantrum because the supermarket (full of food) is an environment where it's likely to happen. Bearing in mind that some of the most common issues that cause children to act out in hostile ways include hunger, tiredness and boredom, make sure they have just eaten and are well rested before hitting the supermarket.

It's also sensible to break up the shopping so that you conquer it in sections. Get your fruit and vegetables from your local fruit shop, your meat from your local butcher, and your staples from one of the supermarket chains. The amount of money you can save by shopping at one of the discount retail or wholesale chains is incredible. Sure, you might not get the same variety in product choice but it makes the shopping experience a whole lot easier when you don't dither between sixteen different brands of the same food. When you are comparing different varieties of the same food, make sure to check the price per 100 grams or 100 millilitres because this will enable you to determine the most cost-effective option.

It is important to only go shopping *after* eating a meal (preferably after breakfast, which is the biggest and most important meal of the day – more to come on this). This applies to both you and your kids, if you have them. The last thing you want is them causing a scene in the supermarket because they're hungry. Going to the supermarket after eating will also prevent those impulse buys that we are inclined to make when we visit the grocery store hungry. It's never the best feeling when you find yourself at the checkout chowing down on that packet of chips or chocolate bar before you've even left.

Most of the shopping can be done on the fringe or outside section of the supermarket, which is where all the fresh produce is located. Although, as I've mentioned, be wary of the ends of aisles, where brands pay to have their products located. There are several aisles that can be skipped altogether, which are loaded with pre-packaged and processed foods that offer very little nutrition. Skip the 'health food' aisle, the chips, the confectionary and the pre-packaged products when you're at the supermarket, so that you won't be tempted by them inside the house. It's much easier than being haunted by a block of chocolate, night after night.

What are considered 'treat' foods?

The following foods (these are just some examples and not an exhaustive list) need to be kept in the 'treat' basket of once per week in the weight-loss months. This doesn't mean you can have all these food items! It means you need to select your favourite. Don't worry, because the great news is you can have them more often during the weight-maintenance months.

Treats

- chips
- biscuits
- snack bars, energy bars or muesli bars
- lollies
- chocolate
- dried fruit
- white bread
- soft drink
- savouries and pastries
- ice-cream
- cakes (this includes banana bread – that stuff isn't healthy just because it's called banana bread. It's the same as having a slice of cake!)

Anything processed or in the confectionary aisle should be thought of as a treat food. Clever marketing and misleading food packaging make things confusing, so be mindful that just because something is labelled 'health food', 'gluten-free', 'dairy-free', 'wheat-free' or 'vegan' doesn't mean it is better for you. It will still be loaded with added sugar and fat and needs to be thought of as a treat.

The reasons for including the foods on this list are many but predominantly because they are very low in nutrition (or have no nutrition) and/or packed full of empty calories. The term 'empty calories' refers to calories that don't provide nutrition. Some of the foods, such as chocolate, are associated predominantly with times of comfort. Even if you are opting for a more nutritious chocolate option – one with greater than 70 per cent cocoa content – it still needs to be in the treat basket. Most concerning is that it's one of those foods we reach for very commonly after dinner when we sit down to relax, only to devour an entire block with ease (I'm going to help you address this later in the book).

Are meal-delivery services any good?

The quick answer is no. But if you're cashed up and time poor, you could consider pre-packaged meals that are delivered to your door or a meal-delivery service that sends you different ingredients and recipes to cook for the week. They are certainly the current fad and it means you don't have to think about what's for dinner. But there's a catch! People become bored of it, just as they do with all commercial programs and products, and end up going back to their old habits when they come off it. These programs are also expensive, don't really help you develop cooking skills or recipes of your own and have a lot of packaging.

More importantly, these programs that you see marketed on your TV, that sell pre-prepared meals and promise the 15 kilogram weight loss in 12 weeks, are based on anecdata (information based on personal experience or observation rather than systematic research and science) – people lose weight and then regain it when they get bored of the program. There is no research to their claims, but clever marketing campaigns would make you believe otherwise.

Shopping for yourself is always going to be more satisfying, nutritionally balanced and importantly will generate less packaging, which is good for the environment.

To avoid being overwhelmed on your first visit to the supermarket on the IWL plan, the following list can form the basis of your grocery shopping going forward. Keep a good supply of these foods in your kitchen, and when they start to run low make sure you add them to your shopping list before they run out. This list can be tailored based on your preferences or dislikes (for example, if you don't like corn, don't buy it) and food-eating practices such as veganism. The most important thing to bear in mind is that each meal you cook will need to include plenty of salad or vegetables, as well as a wholegrain carbohydrate, a source of protein and a source of fat.

Don't be overwhelmed by this list; many of these items are staples that last for a long time, and for those who are beginners or have limited cooking skills, they can be accumulated gradually, as your confidence with cooking develops.

Shopping list

Beverages

- [ ] black tea
- [ ] coffee
- [ ] green tea
- [ ] variety of herbal teas

Condiments, sauces and pastes

- [ ] balsamic vinegar
- [ ] fish sauce
- [ ] honey
- [ ] minced garlic, ginger and chilli (all natural, with vinegar only, and only as a back-up to fresh sources)
- [ ] kecap manis (Indonesian sweet soy sauce)
- [ ] lemon juice
- [ ] lime juice
- [ ] maple syrup

☐ miso paste
☐ ready-made salt-reduced vegetable/chicken/beef stock
☐ red wine vinegar
☐ soy sauce
☐ tahini paste (hulled or unhulled)
☐ wholegrain mustard
☐ 100 per cent nut butter (for example, cashew, peanut or almond)

Dried herbs and spices

☐ basil
☐ black pepper
☐ chilli flakes
☐ cinnamon
☐ coriander
☐ cumin
☐ dill
☐ mixed herbs
☐ mustard seeds
☐ oregano
☐ paprika
☐ salt
☐ thyme
☐ turmeric

Dried goods

☐ baking powder
☐ breadcrumbs
☐ couscous
☐ cornflour
☐ egg noodles

- [ ] rice (basmati, brown, arborio)
- [ ] rice noodles (vermicelli)
- [ ] sugar
- [ ] unsalted dry-roasted or raw nuts
- [ ] variety of seeds (sunflower, flaxseed, pumpkin, sesame)
- [ ] various types of pasta (including wholemeal and wholegrain)
- [ ] wholemeal flour (plain and self-raising)
- [ ] variety of wholegrains such as whole barley, buckwheat, bulgur, freekeh, oats, quinoa (but there are plenty more to choose from – see the list on page 85 – and it is important to try a variety to see what you prefer)

Frozen food

- [ ] mixed berries
- [ ] edamame beans
- [ ] filo pastry
- [ ] frozen vegetables (all varieties)

Fruits and vegetables

all types

Long-lasting vegetables

- [ ] garlic
- [ ] ginger
- [ ] onions
- [ ] potato
- [ ] pumpkin
- [ ] sweet potato

Oils

- [ ] extra-virgin olive oil
- [ ] cold-pressed canola oil

Perishables

- [ ] eggs
- [ ] milk
- [ ] yoghurt (no added sugar) or Greek-style yoghurt
- [ ] wholegrain bread
- [ ] fish
- [ ] meat

Tinned or jarred food

- [ ] beetroot
- [ ] black beans
- [ ] brown lentils
- [ ] cannellini beans
- [ ] capers
- [ ] corn
- [ ] chickpeas
- [ ] chargrilled capsicum strips
- [ ] fish (tuna or salmon in spring water or olive oil)
- [ ] lentils
- [ ] olives
- [ ] pineapple
- [ ] red kidney beans
- [ ] three-bean mix
- [ ] tomatoes
- [ ] low-salt tomato paste

To elaborate on the foods included on this shopping list they are best broken up into several categories including fruits and vegetables, wholegrain carbs, lean protein, healthy fats, snacks and spreads, and condiments.

Fruits and vegetables

There are no bad fruits or vegetables. Despite what you might have been told, bananas and potatoes don't make you fat. They are fine to eat and are, in fact, key weapons in your weight-loss arsenal. They are packed with vitamins, minerals and fibre (both soluble and insoluble fibre, and resistant starch). Insoluble fibre is found in the skin of fruits and vegetables and helps keep your bowel movements regular. Soluble fibre is found in the flesh of fruits and vegetables and helps lower your bad cholesterol (LDL-cholesterol) level by mopping it up and removing it from the blood. And those potatoes that we all fear – well, they are high in resistant starch. The trick is to cook them and then allow them to cool before eating; that way they are packed with resistant starch. This is another type of fibre, which has a prebiotic effect, meaning it promotes plenty of those good bacteria and microbes in the gut that everyone likes to talk about. Of course, there are plenty of other great sources of these three types of fibre, such as wholegrain breads and cereals, pasta, nuts and seeds, lentils, peas and beans, but what I am highlighting is that all of those foods you might fear are actually the ones you need plentiful amounts of. Without them, you will put on weight and you are putting your health at long-term risk.

It's a common story to hear of someone's avoidance of certain fruits and vegetables due to the fear of sugar. The 'sugar-free' movement is confusing and not based on scientific evidence – this is also just anecdata. Many of the sugar-free recipes that you see on the internet still contain sugar, but they are cleverly disguised as expensive sugar alternatives such as rice malt syrup (by the way, the same companies that flog the sugar-free weight-loss programs often also sell these ingredients). Advocates for sugar-free diets say to avoid table sugar, some natural sweeteners such as maple syrup and honey, sweets, berries, condiments and a selection of fruits – an arbitrary list of foods to avoid which has no substance to its claim. Followers of any form of restrictive diet will only obsess about their eating habits in the fear that they will eat something that's not allowed. Inadvertently, what you end up with is a dieting mentality and a cultural obsession with weight loss and body image.

Many of the foods that are blacklisted on sugar-free diets contain naturally occurring sugars. These foods are good for our health as they are packed with fibre. Yes, we need to reduce our consumption of sugar but this needs to happen by reducing our intake of processed foods such as sweets, bakery goods, soft drinks, cakes and chocolate. This doesn't mean reducing your consumption of any fruits or vegetables that contain naturally occurring sugars. These foods are protective for your health; they help prevent heart disease, type 2 diabetes and cancer, and should be part of your daily eating plan.

Wholegrain carbs

Wholegrain carbohydrates are another great source of nutrition, rich in fibre and packed with vitamins and minerals. You should focus on including a source of wholegrain carbohydrates with each meal. Wholegrains, or foods made with them, contain all components of the original grain seed (i.e. the bran, endosperm and germ). All of these must be present to qualify as a wholegrain.

Wholegrains do not include grains such as couscous, white pasta and white rice, and therefore these grains should not be as prevalent in your daily eating plan as their wholegrain cousins. Typically, a wholegrain will be evident on an ingredients list when it has the word 'whole' in front of it, but some forms of wholegrain, such as amaranth, buckwheat, bulgur, freekeh and oats are invariably wholegrain.

Wholegrains include:

- wholegrain or dark rye bread
- wholegrain pasta
- brown rice, also black, purple or red rice
- wild rice
- amaranth
- whole or hulled barley, avoid pearled
- buckwheat
- bulgur
- whole corn
- einkorn
- whole farro/emmer, avoid 'pearled'
- freekeh
- whole khorasan Kamut
- kaniwa
- millet
- oats (any variety is fine, but it is preferable to stick to steel cut or whole rolled oats, because they are less processed)
- quinoa
- whole rye
- whole sorghum
- whole spelt
- teff
- triticale
- whole wheat

Some of these are obscure and hard to find. Don't waste precious time trying to track them down, especially if you live somewhere with limited shopping options. Just stick to brown rice or wholegrain bread.

Bread

Bread is a dietary staple for many of us and with all the choice available nowadays, there is one that is suitable for every lifestyle – the range is exhaustive: wholegrain, multigrain, wholemeal, sourdough, rye, white, high-fibre white, low-GI, gluten-free. It is crucial to include a form you can tolerate, especially because bread is a good source of folate, which is particularly important during pregnancy because it is needed for the growth and formation of the baby's neural tube in the first few weeks. The neural tube forms the brain and spinal cord, and without enough folate the tube doesn't fuse properly, which will cause a neural-tube defect such as spina bifida. Iodine is also needed for the development of your baby's brain and nervous system. It is now a legal requirement that all bread-making flour contains iodised salt (for thyroid health) and folate (a B vitamin), but organic breads are exempt from this rule.

White bread is refined – the bran and germ have been removed – and so is of low nutritional value and not something you should put in your body except as a treat.

Wholemeal bread is made from wholegrains that have been milled to a fine texture, which gives it a plain brown appearance. It contains more nutrition than white but is not the choice to opt for either. Multigrain is not to be confused with wholegrain. Multigrain is made from white flour but has grains added back in. Leave multigrain on the shelves and go for a wholegrain bread instead.

Wholegrain has the entire grain present in the bread – the bran (outer layer), endosperm (starchy middle layer) and germ (nutrient-rich inner part). Wholegrain bread has a dense wholemeal flour base with grains and seeds. Soy and linseed bread is a variety of wholegrain bread with added healthy omega-3 fats.

And then there's rye and sourdough bread. Wholegrain rye bread is the best of the rye choices, but light rye is still better than white bread. The same applies for sourdough – a wholegrain sourdough is the best choice of the sourdough breads. Authentic sourdough (made without yeast and utilising another starter instead) can be quite expensive because it takes a long time to produce and results in an acidic and quite chewy or tough bread.

When it comes to gluten-free breads, they are suitable for those diagnosed with coeliac disease, but they are not healthier than regular breads for the rest of us. They are made with alternative grains to wheat, to avoid the wheat protein, gluten.

The general rule of thumb is to buy wholegrain bread, a wholegrain rye bread, or an authentic sourdough. The occasional wholegrain pita bread to use for wraps is also not going to hurt you (we love making wraps in our household). Ensure the words 'whole wheat' or 'whole wheat flour' is the first ingredient on the label and that 'wholegrain' is high in the ingredient list. Buy the bread that is darkest in appearance and full of grains. Better still, take a visit to your local baker and purchase from there. They are usually very receptive to discussing your specific dietary requirements. A good tip is to keep bread in the freezer and to just get out what you need when you need it.

Coeliac disease is an auto-immune disorder triggered by the consumption of gluten; a protein found in wheat, rye and barley, to give products such as bread their elasticity and texture. But it only affects 1 per cent of the population. When people with coeliac disease eat gluten, they damage their small intestine and can't absorb nutrients from food. They end up with unpleasant side effects such as itchy skin, heartburn, diarrhoea, bloating and constipation. Gluten is not dangerous for the other 99 per cent of us, and cutting it out might do more harm than good because you may be missing out on a rich source of fibre. Despite this, recent research shows the number of people following a gluten-free diet has tripled in the past 10 years. And 70 per cent of those are not diagnosed with coeliac disease, but simply choose to join this trendy movement without properly understanding it, or self-diagnosing symptoms that might be gluten intolerance – or something else entirely.

The only way to determine whether you have coeliac disease is to be tested by your doctor. They might send you for a blood test in the first instance, but the gold standard test is to have an endoscopy, which is where a specialised doctor (a gastroenterologist) sticks a tube down your throat with a camera on it, to examine the lining of your intestine. Self-diagnosing yourself after a chat with friends or colleagues or by taking a quiz online is the worst thing you can do. And stop jumping onto Dr Google – it's doing more harm than good. If you haven't been diagnosed with coeliac disease but are still convinced that you suffer from a gluten intolerance, make appropriate dietary changes, with a focus on including plenty of grains that are naturally gluten-free.

Here are five reasons you shouldn't go gluten-free without a good reason.

1. You will put on weight.

So many of my patients have told me they have removed gluten from their diet because they think it makes them fat. They cut the carbs and then get excited because they see the number on the scales going down. But if you take this option, all you are doing is setting yourself up for a lifetime of misery. Every gram of carbohydrate – which is stored as glycogen in the body – binds three times its weight in water. Therefore, what you see on the scales isn't a decrease in fat mass, but rather a decrease in water content in the body. Wholegrain carbs are the very foods that will help you on your weight-loss journey, not hinder it. Worse still, if you start to include gluten-free biscuits, crackers and other packaged foods in your diet, you will end up putting on weight.

2. You won't get enough fibre.

Wheat, rye and barley are rich sources of fibre, and we need lots of fibre for good bowel health and prevention of heart disease. Unless you make suitable dietary switches, you won't get the necessary 25 grams (females) to 30 grams (males) of fibre that you need every day. Suitable wholegrains that are naturally gluten-free and that are also rich in fibre include rice, quinoa, millet and amaranth.

3. You will feel tired all the time.

Many of my patients also blame gluten for their fatigue and low energy, but there is no evidence that gluten makes you feel sluggish. Instead, the opposite applies. A side effect of any sort of low-carb diet is fatigue and weakness, particularly while exercising. Cutting out the breads and cereals will result in depleted muscle glycogen stores, and without these stores you are going to feel less energetic during moderate and high-intensity exercise.

4. You will increase your risk of cancer.

Everything you have ever been told about gluten causing cancer is false. The only people at risk are the 1 per cent of the population that have coeliac disease. Those gluten products that you are cutting from your diet are high in fibre. Research has clearly proven that a diet rich in wholegrain carbs and cereal fibre – such as breads and cereals – will reduce, not increase, your risk of developing colon cancer.

5. **You will waste your money.**
   Opting for pre-packaged gluten-free products is expensive – many are double the price of the regular version. These products are also higher in fat, salt and sugar, and lower in protein and fibre, than their regular counterparts, in order to make them more palatable. If you are diagnosed with coeliac disease, stick to foods that are naturally gluten-free – fruits, vegetables, dairy, meat, fish, nuts and eggs.

Pasta

Preferably opt for wholegrain pasta, but any pasta is fine, because the focus of any pasta dish needs to be meal balance. You should eat pasta with an accompanying salad so that half of your portion is the pasta and the other half the salad.

Cereal

Buy oats or natural muesli, or oven-bake a large batch of your own muesli that you can use throughout the week (see page 279). When you are in the cereal aisle, avoid all the processed cereals with added sugar – they will leave you starving by 9am.

Rice

Include plenty of brown rice and, if you can afford it, black rice. Basmati rice is also fine and is better suited to some dishes. Also consider alternative grains such as quinoa or barley, but don't feel you have to include them if you don't like them, can't find them or can't afford them. Black rice is delicious but is double the price of brown rice and doesn't suit all dishes.

Lean protein

As a nation and across the Western world we have become fixated on protein, but too much can be detrimental to your health and lead to weight gain. You should include a source of lean protein at each meal but the whole meal shouldn't be protein and you shouldn't be sipping on protein shakes or any form of protein drink or snack post-workout.

There are plenty of lean sources of protein that are suitable to have on your IWL plan. For example, chicken or turkey breast, or other cuts without the skin, 'heart smart' mince, or lean cuts of beef. It is simply a personal preference as to whether you have grain-fed or grass-fed; there is no compelling evidence that grass-fed is significantly more nutritious than grain-fed beef, even though they differ in several nutrients.

The cheaper cuts of meat – like blade or porterhouse – from cattle tend to be the toughest and these are best for slow-cooked dishes where the protein breaks down over time to give it its tenderness. This is fine and makes a difference only to your wallet and method of cooking.

Lamb is a great alternative to beef and packed full of flavour, but unless you can afford the premium cuts, it is a much fattier meat. For example, lamb chops, which you should keep to eating just once per fortnight.

Save pork to a maximum of once per week, because it often comes processed, such as bacon, and is a much fattier meat alternative to beef and lamb. If you enjoy it, opt for lean pork.

Lastly, keep processed meats such as sliced meats, chorizo or salami to the 'treat' category, because they are preserved with additives and salt to prolong their shelf life.

It is easy to pick out the leanest cuts of meat as they will have less marbling or white fatty tissue visible. The white part is the fat.

For meat-lovers, there is no reason every meal needs to be meat. Try reducing your meat consumption to three days per week and include more vegetarian-based options. Including legumes, eggs or tofu is a nutritionally sound alternative to help you achieve your goals on the weight-loss months. For those who don't eat meat, include plenty of legumes (including lentils), eggs and tofu. These are suitable meat alternatives that are also rich sources of nutrition.

Eggs

If you're wondering whether you need to limit eggs, the answer is no! For decades we were told that dietary cholesterol is bad for us. It was thought that the cholesterol found in eggs increased the cholesterol in our blood.

Cholesterol is produced naturally by the liver because it has several vital functions in the body including the production of new cells and hormones that help the body function properly. Therefore, if you don't get enough from your diet, your body will naturally produce it. It needs it to survive. But the reverse also applies. When you consume dietary sources of cholesterol, such as eggs, your liver produces less.

Eggs are a nutritious food, and filling up on wholesome and nutritious foods will help displace less-healthy choices in the diet;

they will *not* increase the bad cholesterol level in the blood. Eggs are a great source of protein and micronutrients that are important for eye and heart health, healthy blood vessels and healthy pregnancies. But I'm not giving you open permission to sit down to a plate of eggs and bacon at every meal. They should be eaten boiled, poached or scrambled, and if fried they should be cooked in a small amount of olive oil.

Seafood

Fish is a great source of protein and fat. You should include plenty of fish and seafood with at least three meals per week. This guideline is the same during pregnancy. However, pregnant women, women planning a pregnancy and children up to the age of six should stay clear of raw fish and top-of-the-food-chain predatory fish: shark (often sold as fish and chips at your local fish shop), kingfish, tuna, king mackerel, orange roughy, ling, swordfish, barramundi gemfish and marlin. These types of fish are all high in mercury, and an unborn baby is most sensitive to the effect mercury can have on their nervous system. Fish take up mercury from streams and oceans as they feed, so the bigger and older they are, the more mercury they will contain. If you do happen to eat one of these types, don't panic, a one-off is not going to affect the health of your baby. All shellfish are nutritious and you can include any type – even shellfish such as prawns are an excellent food source as long as they're properly cooked. Despite everyone's worry about prawns containing cholesterol, shellfish won't increase the cholesterol level in the blood, unless you're eating them covered in batter.

Is farmed or wild-caught better?

Let's take salmon, for example. Nowadays much of the salmon you buy isn't caught in the wild (i.e. oceans, rivers or lakes) but instead bred in fish farms. In fact, globally, approximately 50 per cent comes from fish farms. Farmed salmon has a completely different diet (processed fish feed) to wild salmon (various invertebrates). Nutritionally, yes there are differences, such as there being more fat and specifically more saturated fat in farm-fed versus wild-caught, but the differences are too small to worry about. Due to the high density of fish in fish farms, they are more susceptible to infection and disease than wild fish. To counter this problem, antibiotics are added to fish feed, but this is tightly regulated in developed countries, and not of concern. If you can afford to buy wild-caught Atlantic salmon, then sure, go for this option, but farmed salmon is also perfectly fine and it's what you're going to find in Australia. It's also the choice when it comes to salmon for our household.

And, of course, there are also the patients who ask me about microplastics (very small pieces of plastic that pollute the environ-ment) and the potential harm this can have on their health from consuming wild fish. Research suggests that microplastics are not significantly absorbed by marine life and therefore their potential to accumulate in tissues, and be a problem to our health is very low. It also means they can't be passed on in any significant way to a predator that eats the fish. This, therefore, puts microplastics in a different category to toxic substances, such as mercury, that end up in the food chain from consumption of the internal tissues of fish.

We could discuss the differences between farm-fed and wild-caught fish all day. But as with everything relating to the IWL plan, you don't need to worry about the small stuff. Instead, the emphasis should be on regularly including fish in your IWL eating plan. Don't get caught up in the nitty-gritty detail of whether farmed or wild-caught is better – just make sure you include a variety of fish in your eating plan. For example, you can include salmon on a weekly basis but it shouldn't be the only type of fish you eat. At our place, we like sardines (extremely good value and sustainable), whole barramundi or similar on the barbecue, prawns, salmon, whiting, oysters as a treat and mussels. The benefits of eating fish far outweigh any potential negatives.

Healthy fats

Fat is important for many body processes and you need to include a source of fat with every IWL meal to ensure it is balanced. Great sources of fat include avocado, extra-virgin olive oil, nuts and seeds. These are some of nature's best treats.

Oils

There is no shortage of choice when it comes to cooking oils. Oils play an important role in the diet – we use them for baking, frying, salads and marinades. They are also a source of fat, which is essential for production of cells and hormones, as well as helping the body absorb nutrients. They come in two forms – solid (saturated fat) or liquid (unsaturated fat).

Let's kick it off with coconut oil, because I know you're dying to ask. This has been one of the best marketing scams of the 21st century, although it's a close race between alkaline water, goji berries and almond milk. Coconut oil, much like alkaline water, goji berries and almond milk, should not be part of your diet.

Coconut oil is about 80 per cent saturated fat, so it's solid at room temperature. Government nutrition guidelines tell us to avoid coconut oil because of its detrimental effect on heart health – specifically the fact that it has been shown to raise our low-density lipoprotein (LDL) – otherwise known as our 'bad' cholesterol – which blocks our arteries and causes heart attacks. There are unsaturated oils that can improve your heart health, so you shouldn't be putting this white gunk in your body. Replacing sources of saturated fat with unsaturated fat will reduce your risk of heart attack.

Olive oil is also very popular and a key part of the Mediterranean eating plan. It is obtained from the fruit of olive trees. Whether it be extra-virgin, virgin, pure or light, all varieties of olive oil tick the box when it comes to nutrition, but if you can afford it, you should opt for extra-virgin olive oil as the first choice. The Australian olive-oil industry has exceptionally high standards guaranteeing a fresh and best-quality product, compared to an imported one. You really do get what you pay for when it comes to oil.

Olive oil is predominantly unsaturated fat – those fats that reduce the 'bad' cholesterol in the blood. Better still, olive oil is largely made up of monounsaturated fat rather than polyunsaturated fat. Both mono- and polyunsaturated fats are unsaturated and good for us. However, the modern-day Western diet has meant we are getting too much of one specific polyunsaturated fat called omega-6, particularly from other oils and processed foods such as cakes, bakery goods, biscuits and takeaway foods. Too much of it leads to inflammation. However, a diet rich in olive oil and fish will decrease inflammation in the body and improve your health.

Extra-virgin olive oil is the highest quality olive oil you can buy because it is extracted from the first pressing of olives and has not been subjected to temperature during extraction. Therefore, you often see 'cold pressed' on the label. You can use it for everything, but the smoking point – the temperature at which it goes rancid – varies between the different types of olive oil due to the way they have been processed. You should never let the oil smoke when cooking, so if you find yourself in that position, clean the pan, turn down the heat on the stove and start again. If you follow this rule, you can use extra-virgin olive oil for everything – dipping bread, making salads, marinades and dressings, and when cooking or baking. It is best stored in a dark, cool place to preserve its quality and the bottle should state the harvest date – make sure to use it within 12 months of the harvest date. Other varieties of olive oil will be subject to higher temperatures during extraction and therefore contain fewer antioxidants. Anything labelled 'pure' olive oil has been refined and is not 'extra-virgin', and bottles labelled 'light' olive oil are also not 'extra-virgin' – they are simply lighter in flavour, not fat, which you may have been led to believe.

Canola oil (also known as rapeseed oil) is another popular oil that comes from the seeds of the canola plant – the same plants that produce the small, yellow flowers. Much like olive oil, canola is high in monounsaturated fat and makes up a large part of the Nordic diet – another diet, much like the Mediterranean diet, proven to reduce your risk of heart disease. It has a neutral flavour and high smoking point, making it suitable for baking and stir-frying. Its limiting factor is that it's often found in highly refined forms, so it won't pack nearly as many benefits as extra-virgin olive oil. But you can also buy canola oil unrefined or 'cold pressed', which contains a higher content of antioxidants than their refined counterparts. It's also cheaper than olive oil and is the next-best option.

Sunflower and safflower oil have the same nutritional breakdown and are high in omega-6 polyunsatured fats. Recall that even though polyunsaturated fats are good for us, we get too many of them in the modern-day Western diet. It is a versatile cooking oil due to its high smoke point and light taste, which is why it's commonly used for deep-frying, but it's not something you should be putting in your shopping trolley. Research has also shown that oils rich in polyunsaturated fats, such as sunflower oil, produce toxic substances known as aldehydes when heated, which are detrimental to our health.

Just because it has the word 'vegetable' in it doesn't make it a healthy choice. In fact, vegetable oils fall towards the bottom of the list when it comes to what you should choose. This highly processed and refined extraction of various seeds results in a flavourless and odourless oil that can be subjected to high temperatures. This makes it suitable for deep-frying, but much like many of the oils from which it is derived – sunflower, safflower, sesame, peanut, cottonseed, palm – it is going to be high in omega-6 polyunsaturated fat and best left on the shelf.

There are plenty of oils I haven't discussed because you could write an entire book on all the different oils available. So, if I haven't mentioned it, don't use it. Stick to olive and canola as your oils of choice.

The best way to dispose of oil, whether it's used cooking oil or oil in a jar of semi-dried tomatoes or similar, is to create an oil jar under your sink. Tip the used oil into that jar and seal until next time. When the jar is full, throw it in the bin. Pouring it down your sink is not good for the plumbing, nor for the environment.

Dairy

Dairy can be a source of protein and fat, or just protein if you include skim or low-fat dairy. Research has clearly documented that those who include more dairy products in their diet have a lower body weight, better heart health and are better able to manage their weight than those who don't include them. We still don't have a controlled trial telling us whether skim is better than full-fat for our waistline, so until we do, you should stick to skim or no-fat dairy and focus on milk and yoghurt products, and low-fat cottage cheese. Skim has the same nutrition – calcium and protein – as the full-fat variety with half the calories. You can buy no-fat and low-fat yoghurt without added sugar or you can opt for plain yoghurt and add your own sweetness with fruit or honey. Hang on, I can hear you telling me that full-fat dairy is also fine. If you really prefer to stick with full-fat dairy, yes, this is fine too. I'm fairly confident that when we finally get the results of a controlled trial putting full-fat and skim head-to-head it will show that full-fat is not detrimental to our waistline, but for now I'm just telling you what the current science says. What really matters is that you include dairy and that you include it every day – two to three serves per day.

And then there's everyone's favourite: cheese! Indulging in this food needs to be limited to once per week but can be enjoyed in addition to the treats listed earlier in this chapter. Nutritionally, cheese itself is not the problem. The problem is how we include it in our daily eating habits. Cheese is often one of those foods we cut up and snack on as we prepare the evening meal, only to devour an entire day's calorie intake in a one-hour sitting. It's also something we tend to eat a lot of without noticing. For example, here in Australia when you go to a dinner party or a get-together with friends, cheese is often served before the meal, and you tend to graze on it as you chat. You need to go easy at these times, so it's best to ensure you don't arrive at the dinner party hungry.

To limit your cheese intake, you need to look to other pre-dinner food options that contain the same nutrition but half (or possibly even less than half) the calories. Nuts are a great snack alternative, particularly if you are required to shell them before eating as it slows down your consumption. You could also get stuck into some homemade hummus or beetroot dip with some chopped up vege-tables such as carrot and cucumber, or wholegrain crackers.

What if you avoid dairy?

Nowadays, there's a type of milk for every lifestyle, with milk options (just like cooking oils) taking up nearly a whole aisle in the supermarket. Gone are the days when the biggest decision was deciding between full-cream or low-fat. Instead, now we wander the supermarket deciding between soy milk, A2 milk, rice milk, oat milk, coconut milk, almond milk – not to mention all the other types of nut milk. This brings me to the one thing that stands out when I am lucky enough to travel throughout Europe. Things are simple. There is no plethora of choice. In fact, they scowl – or laugh – if you order an almond-milk latte or soy cappuccino. You get full-cream milk and if you're lucky, low-fat milk. You certainly won't find all the nut-based milks that are the latest fad here. And you might find the same thing in country Australia – I dare you to order a skim almond piccolo latte in the desert!

Whether it be full-cream, low-fat or skim-milk, all varieties of cow's milk tick the box when it comes to nutrition. Cow's milk has eight to nine times the protein content of nut milks and is also a rich source of calcium and vitamin D for healthy bones, and iodine for healthy thyroid function and weight control. The only difference between full-fat and skim is the energy content, because the fat has been stripped off the top, with skim containing half the calories of full-cream milk. However, not everyone can tolerate cow's milk, because it contains lactose – a naturally occurring sugar. Those who are unable to digest lactose (in fact, up to two-thirds of the population) suffer from gastrointestinal side effects such as diarrhoea and bloating. They can still tolerate a splash of milk with their coffee or tea, but they can't sit down to a whole milkshake without side effects. People from Asia are also often lactose intolerant. Lactose-free milk is a suitable option for those who are lactose intolerant because the lactase sugar has been removed from the milk. Nutritionally, it is the same as regular cow's milk.

One of the fastest-growing milk brands is A2. Cow's milk contains both the A1 and A2 milk proteins. Some breeds of cow only produce the A2 milk protein, which is the product you see on the shelves called A2 milk. There is no nutritional difference between the products, but A2 milk will cost you double the price. If you can afford it and prefer it, then great, but there is no reason you need to opt for it. The A1 milk protein is certainly not detrimental to your health and it's likely that anyone who experiences fewer gastrointestinal side effects from drinking A2 milk will also experience the same benefits when drinking lactose-free milk. It's also a fun dinner fact to know that A2 milk still contains a percentage of A1 milk protein (albeit small), so don't think you're skipping the A1 milk protein by guzzling the A2 variety.

Then there's the milk alternatives that are growing in popularity. Almond milk would have to be one of the most talked about products in the 21st century, alongside coconut oil. Almond milk is made by grinding almonds and adding water. It's a rich source of calcium but very low in protein because the actual percentage of almond in the milk is so low. It comes at a high cost due to its production cost and it will contain other ingredients such as stabilisers, emulsifiers and sometimes vegetable oils. Almond milk, or any type of nut milk, is not what we should include in our daily food plan and it's certainly not an appropriate milk substitute for infant formulas, or toddlers or children as they are growing up. Some brands will also be sweetened with added sugar. Almond milk is also devastating for the environment, because of the huge volume of water required to cultivate almonds. Other very popular varieties include oat milk, coconut milk and rice milk. Oat milk is made from whole oats but will also contain other ingredients such as sunflower oil. It's higher in carbohydrate than other milks and therefore will have a small fibre content, but milk is not something we typically source our fibre from. With respect to its protein and calcium content, it stacks up pretty well; it has half the protein of cow's milk, which is much higher than all the different types of nut milk, and the majority of brands will be calcium fortified.

Coconut milk is high in saturated fat, contains no protein and is very low in calcium. It also comes at a high cost. Coconut products are certainly very popular, but the evidence doesn't stack up when it comes to their inclusion in the diet.

Rice milk is made from whole brown rice and other ingredients such as sunflower oil. This is another popular milk hitting our cafes and supermarket shelves. But it's very low in protein – the same as nut milk – and very low in calcium. However, you will find calcium-fortified rice milk on the supermarket shelves.

And then there's soy milk. Soy milk is a liquid extract of soybeans. Unlike all the other milk alternatives, this one actually gets a tick of approval. It is a very popular cow's-milk substitute and unlike all the other dairy alternatives, it matches up for calcium and protein content. This is the one you should choose if you need to avoid cow's milk. Just make sure to buy the 'calcium-fortified' or 'calcium-enriched' product. The one thing that is lacking in soy when compared to cow's milk is iodine – which is needed to manage your weight – and large amounts of soy combined with inadequate intake of iodine can also exacerbate iodine deficiency. Don't get caught up in all that hype about soy being detrimental for your health; it's not true.

Snacks and spreads

Include plenty of:

- nuts (a mix of tree nuts and peanuts, natural or dry roasted, and if you buy in bulk make sure to weigh them out to avoid mindless eating)
- seeds (for example, pumpkin, sunflower and sesame seeds)

- wholegrain crackers
- avocado
- peanut butter (100 per cent peanuts) or any other form of nut butter (for example, cashew butter or almond butter)
- fruit spread (no added sugar)
- Vegemite

How many nuts can you have?

Nuts are one of those foods that we tend to stay away from because of the F word: fat. Even though we know the fat in certain foods such as nuts and seeds is good for us we still hold back because of our fear of fat. This is because we continue to cling to the low-fat weight-loss message that came out in the 1980s, despite it since being dispelled; coupled with the low-fat marketing that we still see on an abundance of supermarket products. It is a difficult field to navigate, which has only resulted in confusion.

Nuts are high in fibre, protein, antioxidants, vitamins and minerals. They are also packed with good-for-you unsaturated fats. This good source of fat, filling fibre and protein found in nuts means your hunger is satisfied for longer. Not only will you enjoy the increased feeling of fullness from nuts but they speed up your metabolism and you don't absorb all the calories when you eat them – in fact, 20 per cent of the energy from nuts is not absorbed at all.

You should have a handful every day – at least 30 grams. This is the amount that can significantly reduce your risk of developing heart disease (by up to 50 per cent) and type 2 diabetes (by up to 27 per cent). But 95 per cent of the population fail to do this. The even better news is that research has shown that up to 3.5 times this quantity (yes, 105 grams!) does not have an adverse effect on a person's body weight when part of a dietary prescription in which nuts replace other calories (such as sweets, bakery goods or takeaway foods).

The health benefits relate to all varieties of nuts, so include a mixture of tree nuts – almonds, walnuts, brazil nuts, cashews, hazelnuts, macadamias, pecans and pistachios. You can also include peanuts, which are classified as a legume and grown underground. But, be careful because you often find yourself having to wade through the many varieties of roasted nuts baked in oil, sugar and salt these days to get to the natural product. These energy-dense and less-nutritious versions of nuts should be avoided. Opt for unsalted varieties and those that are in their raw, natural or dry-roasted form, because these varieties have the same nutrition without the wasted calorie addition.

And lastly, don't buy into the 'activated' scam. Activated nuts are soaked in water for 24 hours and then dried out again so they're still crisp. Despite the clever marketing, there is no research proving that 'activated' nuts are better for you or better for your digestion than natural, raw or dry-roasted nuts. The only change you will notice is the rise in your grocery bill with the additional pricing slapped onto these products.

Butter or margarine?

It's better not to use butter, margarine, or any similar spreads – instead stick to extra-virgin olive oil or avocado as your spread of choice. Some of you might be wondering about those cholesterol-lowering spreads that contain plant sterols. Plant sterols (by the way, we get these from foods such as nuts, seeds, grains and vegetables) work to lower our bad low-density lipoprotein (LDL)-cholesterol levels, but margarines that contain plant sterols need to be consumed in large volumes to get any effect. These are the margarines that you see on television commercials that claim to reduce cholesterol. You need to have 25 grams of a plant sterol margarine spread per day – which equals five slices of bread with 5 grams (or a teaspoon) on every slice – to have a cholesterol-lowering effect.

Condiments

Condiments add flavour to your dish but most of them can be left on the shelf. Stock some low-salt and low-added-sugar tomato sauce, wholegrain mustard, tomato paste, stock cubes or pre-made stock in the fridge; most of the time you will use them in cooking rather than as an accompaniment to the dish.

Condiment consumption should be kept to a minimum or to times when eating out because of their dense-calorie content and minimal nutritional value. This includes mayonnaise, aioli, sweet chilli, Dijon mustard and barbecue sauce. Everyone knows someone who saturates every meal with sauce. I love a condiment too, but you need to be mindful of what you are adding to your plate. For example, for every dollop of sweet chilli sauce you also get 5 teaspoons of sugar, for teriyaki marinade it's nearly 3 teaspoons of sugar, for tomato sauce it's 2.2 teaspoons of sugar, for tomato chutney it's 1.2 teaspoons of sugar and for sriracha (hot chilli) sauce it's about 0.8 teaspoons of sugar. The same rule applies to all those cleverly marketed fat-free or low-fat salad dressings – you must be mindful of how much you add to your meal. You can leave the fat-free and low-fat on the shelves and buy the ordinary full-fat version because the fat-free and low-fat option is likely to be higher in sugar anyway.

The benefits of fermented foods

Your body contains trillions of bacteria that help you stay healthy, the majority found in your intestines or gut. But it's not all good.

Your gut contains both 'good' and 'bad' bacteria and its composition is largely determined by what you feed it. Processed and fast food will increase the number of bad bacteria in the gut, whereas foods high in fibre and fermented foods will increase the amount of good bacteria. Fruit, vegetables and wholegrain carbohydrates are important, as they are rich sources of fibre and contain prebiotics, which acts as a food source for the good bacteria in the gut. So too are milk-based products and foods that have been fermented because these contain probiotics that are live microorganisms or good bacteria and exist in our gut to keep it healthy. Prebiotics are the fuel for probiotics and consequently both are needed to increase the population of healthy bacteria in your body.

When a food is fermented it is left to sit until the sugars that the food naturally contains interact with bacteria, yeast and microbes. This process results in an altered chemical structure of the food. Kimchi and sauerkraut are two such examples that are great to include in your IWL plan – try making your own at home. Kimchi is a staple of the Korean diet, and there's a lot to be said for the Korean diet – they have one of the lowest prevalences of obesity in the world. However, fermented foods are not for everyone due to their strong flavour, aroma, sourness and availability, and you will find the same good bacteria – probiotics – that you find in fermented foods in milk-based products such as yoghurt. By incorporating the foods outlined in the IWL plan (the third principle of the IWL plan – *Full rainbow*) you will improve the bacteria in your gut, which will help you on your weight-loss journey.

The value of canned and frozen foods

Both canned and frozen foods play a vital role in your IWL plan. You should stock your cupboard with tomatoes, lentils, chickpeas, tuna, salmon, fruit in natural juice and some low-salt vegetable soup. Jarred garlic and ginger (no added sugar or salt) are also a practical alternative to avoid relying on fresh produce all the time. However, appreciate that fresh garlic and fresh ginger are much more flavoursome and you can notice the difference in cooking. Again, opt for locally sourced produce to ensure better quality. Also appreciate that at IWL HQ, we often can't be bothered and frequently use the jarred stuff.

In your freezer, you should stock some frozen vegetables, frozen berries or other fruit, and frozen yoghurt. Another food myth that's been around for a very long time is that frozen vegetables and fruit aren't as good for you. They are snap-frozen at the time of harvest and hence retain the same level of nutrients as fresh vegetables. Frozen fruit also allows you to enjoy raspberries and blueberries in the dead of winter and veggies out of season, plus they're often cheaper than their fresh counterparts.

You can also use your freezer as a major meal-prep tool. Produce is cheaper in bulk, so we often buy the largest packet of chicken breasts or salmon, then portion up (avoiding plastic wrap!) into containers and freeze until we need them. In our household, we are also big fans of doubling a meal and eating it for lunch or putting it in the freezer for another time. Fried rice, pasta and risotto all make great freezer meals. Another winner is cooking an entire packet of brown rice when you have the time and freezing.

Beverages and treats

You should stock your cupboard with tea, coffee and sparkling water. A SodaStream can also come in handy at home. Having a soda with fresh lime is a great way to add more fluid to your day, especially if you are not particularly fond of plain old water. Coffee and tea are good for your health but try to stick to no more than two cups per day due to the stimulant effect of caffeine. Also make sure to avoid it after 4pm, because caffeine can disrupt your sleep or ability to fall asleep.

Treats are all those foods that are processed. For example, banana bread, chips, ice-cream, chocolate and biscuits. We all have our favourites and you can (and should!) include them on the IWL plan. Treats must be portion-controlled, so buy chocolates or ice-creams in individual packaging, or divvy biscuits into separate containers to avoid eating the whole packet or tub. As I've already said and will say again, you *shouldn't* cut out any foods on the IWL plan.

Navigating your way when dining out

It can be quite challenging to navigate the food options if you are constantly exposed to lunch meetings and evening functions. If they are unavoidable, you need to be selective about your menu choices and stick with entrée-sized meals as opposed to main-course sizes. Dining out meals are double the energy content of home-cooked meals and are also higher in salt and saturated fat. The chef's job is to make the food tasty so this means extra flavour and taste with liberal amounts of oil, cream, butter, sugar and salt.

Where possible, stay clear of hot food and try to stick to cold food options such as sushi, and cafes with sandwich and salad options. Hot foods like pasta or burgers often feature hidden calories. For those instances where you are not able to select the dining venue, here are a few suggestions for healthy dish choices for different cuisines.

American

Choose salad-based meals but ask for the dressing on the side.

Australian pub food and modern Australian

Opt for salmon or steak. Instead of the hot chips, ask for salad with dressing on the side or steamed/boiled vegetables with no added condiments.

British

Select stand-alone meat- and vegetable-based dishes.

Chinese

Choose vegetable- or fish-based dishes, avoid fried dishes, and share plates with others if possible. Ask for boiled rice instead of fried.

Fast-food road stops

Select pre-made sandwiches or salads. Even though they will contain added condiments that you would otherwise not use at home, this is a much healthier and more nutritious option than burgers, fries or fried chicken.

French

Select dishes such as steamed mussels and salads with vinaigrette dressing.

Greek

Opt for grilled meats and vegetables, fish cooked in tomatoes (plaki), or Greek salad.

Indian

Choose steamed rice and tomato-based dishes. Avoid curries made with coconut milk or cream.

Italian

Select tomato-based pastas (entrée size) or salads. Avoid energy-dense appetisers such as garlic bread.

Japanese

Select sushi or sashimi, miso soup, edamame or seaweed salad. Avoid fried foods.

Korean

Try different varieties of kimchi and bibimbap and avoid fried foods.

Malaysian

Share plates with others if possible. Opt for salads and steamed rice instead of fried. The general rule is to control portion size and to avoid fried dishes.

Mediterranean

Choose salads and meat-based dishes.

Mexican

Select grilled fish or meat, salsa, jalapenos, chicken or beef fajitas or enchiladas (ask for no cheese and no sour cream).

Thai

Choose a stir-fried dish accompanied by vegetables, or try chilli beef (neua pad prik), and share plates if possible. Avoid fried spring rolls and try fresh spring rolls. Opt for steamed rice instead of fried.

Vietnamese

Opt for rice paper rolls, salads, steamed whole fish, or traditional soups such as pho.

If you find yourself at a buffet, limit your plate to three choices that will satisfy you. If you introduce new foods as you go back to the buffet, you are more likely to overeat.

What about veganism?

More people than ever are turning to veganism for a variety of reasons, including ethical, cultural, environmental and health grounds. Veganism is a type of vegetarian diet that means abstaining from all animal products. This means no meat, poultry or fish. It also means eating no animal by-products such as eggs and dairy products. This eating plan consists of fruit, vegetables, nuts, seeds and legumes and it can be quite challenging to meet your nutritional requirements for a variety of vitamins and minerals. It raises six nutritional alarms.

If you've chosen to go vegan, the first two nutrients you need to consider are calcium and vitamin D. They are both needed for strong bones and to prevent osteoporosis, a disease that leaves you more prone to fractures. The richest source of calcium is dairy. It is also a bio-available source of calcium, meaning this nutrient is highly absorbed in the body. However, if you are avoiding dairy products, opt for calcium-fortified soy products, which are the next closest nutritionally complete alternative. Almonds, dark green leafy vegetables and tofu are also good sources of calcium but their bio-availability is low, meaning you need much more of this food source to meet your recommended nutrient intake. With respect to vitamin D, which helps absorb calcium from the stomach, it is found in by-products of animals including cheese and eggs, and the skin of fish. But the best source is the sun. A supplement may be required if you are not getting a lot of sunlight.

The third nutrient that requires special consideration is iron. Iron helps transport oxygen around the body, so if you're feeling tired when you go on a vegan diet, it's likely your iron levels are low. Menstruating women have a much higher iron require-ment than men – more than double – due to the monthly loss of blood. Meat is a haem (blood) source of iron, meaning it is highly absorbed in the body. There are lots of non-haem sources of iron including dark green leafy vegetables, fortified cereals, kidney beans, chickpeas, lentils and almonds, but just like with calcium you need much more of these plant-based sources to meet your recommended dietary intake. Not much of the iron from the spinach that Popeye eats actually gets into his muscles. Popeye's legendary love for spinach was incorrectly calculated due to a misplaced decimal point. Way back in 1870, a German chemist by the name of Erich von Wolf was researching the amount of iron in spinach. When writing up his research, he mistakenly recorded 35 milligrams of iron in 100 grams of spinach instead of 3.5 milligrams – 10 times more generous than reality. This mistake led to the rise of Popeye and the popular misconception that spinach is exceptionally high in iron, which makes the body stronger.

The fourth is vitamin B12. This vitamin is required for the formation of red blood cells as well as a healthy brain and nervous system. It is only found in animal products – much higher in the animal itself rather than a by-product – and only a tiny amount is required for healthy body function. It is not found in plant sources of food and therefore it is vital to choose fortified foods such as breakfast cereals and soy products – soy milk, tofu and miso. This is one I would recommend getting checked by your general practitioner, because a supplement may be required.

If you ask anyone what fish is good for, they will tell you a healthy brain. Which brings us to the fifth nutrient of concern. This is because fish is a rich source of omega-3 fatty acids, and eicosapentaenoic acid (EPA) and docosahexaenoic acid (DHA) are two crucial ones for brain health. Alpha-linolenic acid (ALA) is the plant-based form of omega-3, which is converted to EPA and DHA in the body. However, not all omega-3 fatty acids are created equal and this conversion process from ALA to EPA and DHA is not overly efficient. Again, you need more of the plant-based source to meet your recommended dietary intake. EPA and DHA are found in fish, while ALA is found in oil, nuts, seeds and vegetables.

The last consideration is iodine. Iodine is essential for a healthy thyroid and this gland is the gatekeeper to our metabolism and a healthy weight. Iodine is found in the earth's soils but farming practices have resulted in iodine-deficient soils, increasing the risk of iodine deficiency. The richest sources of iodine are fish – found in the skin – and dairy products. Plant-based sources include seaweed, wholegrain bread and beans.

Last, but not least, it is important to note that products labelled 'vegan' are not necessarily healthier. Many are highly processed and high in added sugar and fat. The same can be said for 'gluten-free' products. Just because something is devoid of a particular food or nutrient doesn't make it healthier, so beware of clever marketing. It's a bit like the 'clean-eating' con. It's just ingenious marketing to make it appear as though you are eating healthier. Anything that is processed is a 'treat' and must be kept in the occasional pile.

If you are unsure whether you should be taking a calcium, iron, vitamin B12 or vitamin D supplement, consult with your general practitioner who can perform a blood test to check and advise.

There are also other types of commonly followed vegetarian diets. Some can make it easier to meet your nutritional requirements but you can also miss out on one of the six nutrients mentioned above if you avoid certain foods or food groups.

Pescatarian and flexitarian are two varieties of vegetarian diet that are growing a greater following as people choose to move away from eating meat all the time. A pescatarian will avoid meat and allow fish. A flexitarian will only occasionally eat meat, for example, a couple of times per week. It is unlikely you are at risk of any deficiencies if following this type of eating pattern.

And then there is the lacto-ovo category of vegetarian diets. Lacto-ovo vegetarians include dairy products and eggs but not meat; lacto vegetarians include dairy products but not eggs or meat; and ovo vegetarians include eggs but not dairy or meat. It is important that suitable substitutions are made to your IWL plan if you are following one of these types of vegetarian diets.

Your task

Throughout this chapter I have provided a list of the foods to include on the IWL plan, as well as a list of foods you can snack on between breakfast, lunch and dinner, and a shopping list. Write down these lists or photocopy the pages and keep them on the fridge, so they are visible every time you visit the kitchen. There are also downloadable versions of these lists at intervalweightloss. com.au.

CHAPTER 9

THE FOURTH PRINCIPLE: USE CHOPSTICKS

Before I explain the significance of the fourth principle of the IWL plan – *Use chopsticks* – I want to reflect on something I have already mentioned but deserves special attention to help you better understand how the IWL plan works. Over the past few decades the level to which we have become fixated on meal plans and calorie counting has become evident. This comes back to the dieting mentality and being brainwashed to believe that if we sit down, count calories and follow a set meal plan, we will succeed. Those four-, eight- and 12-week programs are just cleverly marketed and neatly packaged products specifically targeted at women to make you feel like you are getting something for your dollar. Sure, we need structure and we need to plan, but fixating on meal plans only sets you up for failure. Research proves that people don't stick to these plans for more than a couple of months because it's not sustainable.

The IWL plan doesn't require you to sit down and meticulously record every piece of food you put into your body, because not only do you have more important things to do, it makes no difference. It is absurd that these programs have you weighing out specific quantities of food and searching for all sorts of things you have never even heard of, let alone are able to pronounce. For example, sugar. Who cares what sugar you use – there is no nutritional difference between white sugar, brown sugar and any of the other types of sugar. Remember, one of the reasons people easily succeed on the IWL plan is that it's realistic and simple, so it can be easily applied to real life. You don't have to neglect time with the girls or run late for picking up the kids because you were stuck in the supermarket searching for obscure ingredients. It also won't leave you hungry all the time, because as you just learnt with the third principle of the IWL plan – *Full rainbow* – this plan is not about restricting but rather increasing your food intake from wholesome, nutritious foods, leaving you eating more, not less.

The fun of learning how to use chopsticks

Dinner can be a stressful time for many households. Whether it's the one-year-old throwing most of their food on the floor, the children fighting at the table or the complaint that they don't like the food, you still need to make sure everyone sits together, preferably at the dinner table and away from technological distraction. Not only do you need to be mindful of what you are eating but you also need to set a good example by making this a daily ritual. This is especially relevant if you have an infant or toddler, because they pick up things at a very early age.

The best news is that you don't have to cook separate meals for yourself with the IWL plan, and if you have a baby, there are plenty of recipes at the back of the book that you can make and blend for your child. In fact, everyone in the household can enjoy the same food on the IWL plan. Yes, you can still cook all those simple meals that you are used to cooking, such as spaghetti bolognaise; the only difference is the portion sizes. Let the kids eat to their appetite but you need to serve your evening meal on a tiny plate (bread-and-butter size) or a very small bowl (Asian rice-bowl size) and the meal must be eaten with chopsticks. Yes, you read that correctly! The fourth principle of the IWL plan is – *Use chopsticks!* The same applies if your partner or husband is following the plan. They, too, should serve up their evening meal on a small plate and eat it with chopsticks – unless you're a chopsticks master, in which case you should use a teaspoon. Men typically have a bigger body mass, so they often need more food than women. But let them start with a smaller serve than they are used to and go back for seconds by filling up on more salad and vegetables.

So, if you have never learnt to use chopsticks, now is the time. It can be frustrating and difficult at first, but you will eventually get the hang of it. The more uncomfortable you are with them, the better, because this will force you to eat even slower. The whole point of incorporating chopsticks into the evening meal is to slow you down. Don't give up if you don't master chopsticks straight-away. It's quite fun, and if it's a family you're feeding, you'll most likely see them embracing the chopsticks too.

The importance of the chopsticks

Slowing down your meal and serving up less food at the evening meal allows time for signals to be sent from your stomach to your brain to tell you that you are full. We are hardwired to eat huge portions at dinner. Consequently, we don't even give our body a chance to tell us we don't need any more food. The only way to give yourself a chance of listening to your body's cues is by forcing yourself to eat slower, and hence the mandatory use of chopsticks or a teaspoon.

What to do if you're still hungry

Allow your brain the time to gauge its fullness (approximately 10 minutes after eating) and listen to your appetite hormones. If you're still hungry after the first serve, wait 10 minutes before then going back for a second serve. If you are still hungry after your second serve, you are either still eating too quickly (but this is unlikely unless you are a master of the chopsticks), or you simply didn't focus most of your food intake in the morning through to lunch. You may also need to reflect on some common identity excuses such as lack of time and lack of hunger, which are often high on the list. If you do find yourself still hungry, you need to adjust how much food you are eating in the morning to give yourself a chance of eating less at the dinner table. You will never feel hungry in the morning if you over-eat every night, and you will always be time-poor if you devote everything to work and the kids and nothing to yourself. This change can be hard to get used to and won't happen overnight. A lifetime of learned behaviours can take time to break – remember the 66-day rule!

In the actual circumstance where you are hungry because you have messed up your eating for the day – for example, meetings got in the way or you were running late to get to an appointment or to pick up the kids from school (we all have different reasons) – don't panic. In this instance, it is important to have emergency foods surrounding you, such as fruits, dairy products and nuts, so that you don't go and binge on sweets or foods from the vending machine if you are still in the office, or end up at the drive-through if you're playing taxi driver for the kids. If you missed lunch due to meetings, don't panic! This happens to everyone and you will get better at planning around such situations. In this instance, have your lunch at afternoon tea time, wait an hour and then have your afternoon tea, before then sitting down to dinner as the smallest meal.

The goal needs to be making dinner the most important meal from a social and cultural perspective – a time where you sit down at the dinner table and reflect on your day, perhaps writing in a journal as you eat if you live alone. It can also be a time to engage with others if you don't live alone. Conversation will slow your eating, as will writing some notes in a journal. Research has proven that if you can hear yourself eat, it slows your eating pace.

> There is no better way to sum up the IWL plan than from an IWL community member, who said: 'You'll be amazed at how easy this lifestyle is. I haven't eaten like this since I was a skinny teenager & the weight just keeps slowly falling away. Just follow the principles & you too will be amazed.'

Breakfast as the biggest meal of the day

'Eat breakfast like a king, lunch like a prince, and
dinner like a pauper.' – *Adelle Davis*

Research has proven that those who eat breakfast every day are better able to manage their body weight. We have it all wrong in the modern-day Western lifestyle. We wake up, rush out the door, grab a coffee if we can, and then power through the morning only to have our first meal closer to lunch (if we're lucky). We get home from work ravenous, only to reach for anything we can get our hands on, and then dinner ends up being the largest meal of the day. This is the wrong way to orientate your food intake.

Breakfast is the most important meal on the IWL plan, and you must ensure you are well prepared and consuming most of your food in the earlier part of the day. Even if this means you are running out the door with a kid under each arm, you still need to take breakfast with you. It might be a tub of yoghurt with some fruit and nuts, or a Tupperware container of muesli with honey and berries that you prepared the night before. You must then focus on tapering off the volume of food so that lunch becomes the next-biggest meal of the day and dinner the smallest.

Most people struggle with the lack of guidance around portion sizes when first starting out on the IWL plan. Therefore, to help you kickstart the process and to give you something to work with as a guide (I stress, this is a very rough guide that is simply a starting point), breakfast will be a portion size that is equivalent to three closed hand fists, lunch will be two closed hand fists and dinner will be one closed hand fist. This guide excludes vegetables, so you can load up as many vegetables and salad as you like at each meal. Some people will need more – for example, four closed hand fists at breakfast, three at lunch and two at dinner – and others will need less. It is simply a starting point to help kickstart the process. But, as a general rule, you can eat as much as you like at breakfast because as long as you are eating most of your food at breakfast and then cutting down through lunch and making dinner your smallest meal, you are doing well. I never want you to deprive yourself of food, so if you're still hungry after starting with these rough guides, always make sure to go back for more vegetables or salad at each meal.

Your food requirement will increase during pregnancy (particularly during the third trimester) and when breastfeeding. You may need one and a third times the food you typically eat (this is fine and encouraged).

The initial barrier

It is very uplifting when you first read someone's introductory story in the 'Interval Weight Loss Community' Facebook group.

There are a few from people who have never dieted and get it from the very start, but there are many others who fail to grasp the basic principles of the IWL plan. They kick off with all good intentions but find it hard to overcome the fact that the IWL plan doesn't come with set meal plans or a required number of calories to consume. They still have 'dieting' in their head. Straightaway I know this is, sadly, someone who has unknowingly wasted thousands of dollars on a plethora of diets and online weight-loss programs. And in many regards, their fixation with meal plans is simply leftover from a lifetime of dieting. If you are reading this and relate to this common scenario, it is likely you still have 'dieting' in your head. Many don't get past this initial hurdle and then find themselves going back to their old ways, only to follow the same old programs with the same disappointing results. I will help you avoid this situation, but, as previously mentioned, I ask that you re-read this book to instil the principles of the plan.

The problem with meal plans and calorie counting

Ever since the rise of the diet industry we have been brainwashed into thinking the answer is in set meal plans; that the only way to succeed is when we are told exactly what to weigh out and eat. But it's much easier than this, and I will help you move away from the mentality of relying on set meal plans and counting calories. After all, you can't spend the rest of your life on a 12-week program! And it's certainly not adaptable to the rest of the family. It's also likely to have an influence on your kids, because they watch and follow your every step. You don't want them to think dieting is accepted and normal.

Despite what people might think, weight loss is not as simple as calories in versus calories out. The body is far too complex for that and as you have learnt, your body will adjust its metabolic rate based on how much food you feed it. Quite simply, calorie counting is a waste of time and there is nothing to be gained from meticulously recording your calorie intake in a smartphone app. Not only will you find huge errors in some of the reported calories in foods, but more importantly, all calories are different. One classic example is nuts. We don't absorb all the calories (about 20 per cent is not absorbed) when we eat nuts because the cell membranes lock in some of the fat and prevent it from being absorbed. They also increase our resting energy expenditure and they fill us up for long periods of time. So, even though they are a source of fat, albeit a good source of fat, their calorie content is not an accurate reflection of what your body is absorbing. Vegetables are the same, with their high fibre content. A lot of the calories, particularly in uncooked fruit and vegetables, make their way to the large intestine undigested and therefore are not absorbed in the body.

For years we have been told to count calories, to only eat certain foods for breakfast, to avoid carbs at night, and so on. This only compounds the issue. By focusing on the foods that are outlined earlier in this book you will see a reduction in the number of calories you are consuming without even focusing on it. More importantly, you won't feel hungry all the time, like you do on diets, and you will provide your body with the nutrition it needs.

Hunger scale

The following scale is a useful tool to help you with your portion sizes, especially when you are first starting out on the plan. During the wash-out month (a time where you can get used to implementing the IWL plan), you should use a diary to record your hunger scale before and after meals. It is not the actual meal I am interested in you recording but rather what your appetite is doing and how it changes throughout the day.

-1	0	1	2	3	4
Full and uncomfortable	Not at all hungry	Satisfied	Slightly hungry	Somewhat hungry	Hungry

It takes time to gain an appreciation for how your appetite signals work in the body, and this is not something that changes overnight. The 66-day rule applies here too. If you notice that your hunger is high before meals at the end of the day (a '3' or '4' on the hunger scale), you have a few tweaks to make. This is particularly relevant if you have been in the same routine for years – skipping meals, eating little throughout the day and having your biggest meal at dinner. The first step is simply to change your food structure, to ensure you start to wake up hungrier in the morning. Over time, you should start to wake up in the '3' range. If you wake up in the '4' range, you are doing very well.

The scale is also useful for recording your hunger after meals. Most of the time you should feel '1' after eating, rather than '0' or '-1'. When you first start the IWL plan, you will find the evening time the most challenging – the change to a bread-and-butter plate or rice bowl can take some getting used to. I don't want you to deprive yourself of food, so if you are still hungry after your first serve, go back for more. This is especially relevant during pregnancy and when breastfeeding. As discussed, your appetite will increase during these times and this is normal and expected; after all, you are growing and feeding another person.

Before you go back for more, you must apply the 10-minute rule: you should wait at least 10 minutes before serving more food, because this is the time needed for your appetite signalling to work (that is, the time it takes for signals to be sent to your brain telling you whether you need more food). In saying this, you can still eat as much salad and as many veggies as you like, and this applies to all meals. And irrespective of whether you're pregnant or breast-feeding, you still need to follow the 'funnel plan', which is eating progressively smaller meals throughout the day. The only difference is you might need up to one and a half times the quantity of food.

Remembering to eat

The thought of regular eating on the IWL plan can be quite difficult to get your head around after a lifetime of food derivation – the dieting mentality. But believe it or not, one of the biggest challenges towards ensuring success on the IWL plan is *remembering to eat*, and it's a positive remark I often hear from my patients and members of the 'IWL Community' Facebook group.

Food preparation is the key, as discussed in the fourth principle of the IWL plan – *Full rainbow*. If you prepare, you will never need to worry about a common scenario: convenience eating. This is something my patients often complain about – that is, they could never find any good options on the road when driving their kids around. Quite frankly, you won't, and it's just another of those identity excuses I discussed in Chapter 2. The modern-day environment ensures this; there is no shortage of fast food, and it is very challenging to find healthy options on the go. Not to mention the high cost, if you do. You must take food with you as you leave home every day (for you and your kids); this is the only way to ensure success. You must also set alarms on your phone to prompt you to eat and to enjoy the food away from technological distraction. If you take your own food and remember to eat it (even if it's just some fruit and nuts), you will not find yourself looking for emergency food on the go from the drive-through, the corner store or the vending machine. Even if this just means a couple of bites of food when the opportunity arises – it is much better to do this and prevent the hunger pangs creeping in, which only results in reaching for the junk.

Most of your food intake will happen at the start of the day – that is, from breakfast to lunch – and you should always include afternoon tea, perhaps at the same time as the kids or if you're working, before you leave for the day or when commuting home. If you skip a meal or miss one due to a back-to-back work schedule, it will result in hunger, which can in turn result in a downward spiral of food choices and overconsumption. Always have snacks on hand to avoid this situation. It's much better to snack on some fruit or nuts in between meetings or in the car while going to pick up your kid from childcare than it is to find yourself grabbing McDonald's on the way home.

Good snacks that don't take much preparation include a handful of nuts (dry-roasted almonds or cashews are ideal), yoghurt, a piece of fruit, a piece of toast with avocado or nut-based spread, a tin of tuna on wholegrain crackers, some chopped up carrots or cucumber with dip or a pre-cooked packet of brown rice with vegetables. (We roast a whole heap of vegetables on the weekend at IWL HQ and use throughout the week.)

Managing the afternoon stress

The end of the day can be the most challenging. You may be juggling full-time work with kids or you may just lead a very busy work life. Consequently, the thought of the comfortable couch with food and drink in hand is enticing. The same can be said when we associate cooking at the end of the day with winding down and the subsequent snacking and drinking. Often, we attribute this to stress. But as much as we like to, eating and drinking is the last thing we should be doing to de-stress and unwind. This certainly makes us feel good at the time, as we are fulfilling the need for a 'quick fix', but it doesn't feel good the next morning when we wake up with a foggy head or the guilty feeling of poor food choices accompanied with overeating.

If it has been a stressful day, don't jump straight on to the couch or into the cooking when you get home. Instead (work out what's practical for you), go for a walk with the kids or burn out a quick 20-minute exercise session (there are some example sessions provided on pages 159 to 162) to get those endorphins pumping around the body and to alleviate stress. It doesn't matter what the exercise is, all that matters is you address the stress before putting yourself in an environment where you are tempted to self-medicate with alcohol and junk food or high-calorie comfort foods. Cheese and wine are usually high on the list!

Kids' leftovers

It's very tempting to eat your kids' leftovers or to pinch a mouthful of food while they eat, as you don't want to create waste. This form of mindless eating can also be due to many other factors including stress, boredom, hunger and lack of sleep. It's called the 'If it's there, you'll eat it' phenomenon and it can be a challenging habit to break, particularly towards the end of the day. However, the biggest rule you need to impose on yourself relates to not eating your kids' leftovers. Preferably, you should eat at the same time as your kids, but this must be done by serving up your own plate or bowl of food. They will copy your behaviour, so if they see you eating it, they're more likely to eat it themselves. For many reasons, this is not always practical, depending on the ages of your kids, and if this is the case, you should try to eat before serving your kids to ensure you feel satiated. If they do leave leftovers (and they will a lot of the time), cover and put them in the fridge so you can serve them later or throw them out. Of course, it is better to prevent food wastage, and we freeze all our scraps for the neighbouring chooks.

Implementing the IWL plan for shift workers

If you work different shifts, including nights, the IWL plan can be adapted to your lifestyle. The same principles still apply. Yes, it seems strange, but it still applies. There is no question that shift work makes it even harder to manage your weight because it disrupts your circadian rhythm (your body clock), but by following the principles of the IWL plan you are giving yourself the best chance of doing so. Your food intake should always be funnelled down as the day progresses and therefore you need to focus on having your biggest meal when you wake up before you go to work. That time will differ for everyone depending on their shift. For example, if you start work at 9pm and wake up in the afternoon, this would be the time to have your first meal – your breakfast or biggest meal of the day. And then as per the IWL script, your portion sizes should taper off throughout your work shift (i.e. eating less as the day goes on). This will mean that you're sitting down to dinner with your chopsticks at a time that would be breakfast for most. If you regularly change shifts and really don't feel like eating your biggest meal of the day before a night shift, you should still apply all the other IWL principles and ensure to eat regularly to prevent hunger setting in – even if you just grab a couple of bites of food when you can. I'm not going to pretend it's easy for you. It's certainly challenging working shifts but many people who work shifts have the same poor eating habits that we all have – skipping meals, eating most of their food intake at the end of the shift, and frequently consuming takeaway food.

Sophie is an IWL community member and works as a nurse. She tends to do a handful of graveyard shifts in a row each month whereby she will start around 9pm and then finish at 6am. On these days she typically wakes up in the afternoon around 3, will go for a long leisurely stroll first thing to get some natural blue light and then come home to make her coffee and first meal of the day. Sophie would also use this time to cook something she could take to work and have as her dinner after getting home the next day. She would have a snack on the way to work. In an ideal world she would sit down and eat her packed lunch during her break, but because she works in emergency, sometimes it can be manic and on these shifts she just races to the kitchen whenever the opportunity arises for a few bites of food. It might be a mouthful of her packed lunch, some yoghurt, a piece of fruit or a handful of nuts. She would then have a snack in the car on the way home from work and typically this would be something high in fat and natural sugars – nature's treats – to resist the temptation to stop at McDonald's. Her favourites would be avocado or honey on wholegrain toast, which she would make at the end of the shift, or a tub of yoghurt with some berries. If she felt like it, she would eat when she got home from work but on the occasions where she was exhausted, she would make sure to have more food on the way home from work so she could shower and jump straight into bed. Sophie has managed to juggle her different shifts as a nurse. Some days are easier than others but overall she has adapted to the changes well and has managed to successfully lose weight along the way.

Your task

If you don't have any chopsticks, go out and treat yourself to a pair. (A hot tip – chopsticks that often come with takeaway meals can also be used again and again.) Along with this book, they are going to become one of your best friends for life.

CHAPTER 10

THE FIFTH PRINCIPLE: CHOOSE TO MOVE

The ability to walk on two legs is one of the earliest defining human traits and evolved around six million years ago. Movement was needed to survive, and this is still evident in parts of the globe; not only with our remaining hunter–gather tribes but also in modern civilisation. For example, while food – the quality and quantity of it – is often cited as a leading factor in Europeans' comparatively long life expectancy, other lifestyle features also play a role. One of those is that activity is part of everyday life. People don't sit on their bum all day and then drive to the gym. In fact, you will seldom see a gym. Instead, they make movement a priority by walking to and from town and the shops, and to run their errands. Many carry their groceries. They use public transport and make use of cycle paths to bike to and from work. Walking or cycling 15 to 20 kilometres per day is the norm. We, on the other hand, drive everywhere, put the robot vacuum cleaner to work and wait in our living room for the food to be delivered. These technological innovations have solved the physical demands of manual labour but created new challenges for the human body. Take cleaning, for example; the old-school way of cleaning your rug was to bang the bejesus out of it on the balcony for 10 minutes, which burns the equivalent of a cheeseburger (300 calories). On the contrary, turning on the robot vacuum burns nothing.

We evolved to walk long distances and hunt for food, as part of a nomadic lifestyle; not a lifestyle in which we sit in front of screens and turn on gadgets to do the work for us. Our sedentary lives are literally killing us, with one in ten deaths worldwide being attributable to physical inactivity. However, irrespective of your size or your aches and pains, I'm going to help you get moving so that not only will you be active every day, but you will love it. This is the fifth principle of the IWL plan – *Choose to move*. Whenever the opportunity arises, you are going to *choose to move*.

What does the research show?

When it comes to how much exercise we are currently doing, it doesn't bode well. Only one in three people are meeting the measly guideline of two-and-a-half hours of activity per week (30 minutes on five days per week) recommended to keep healthy. Even fewer people do the recommended and additional two days per week of muscle-strengthening exercises – something that will significantly reduce your chances of dying prematurely by a whopping 20 per cent.

Where do you start?

The first step is to get yourself an activity monitor and over the course of a week see how much activity you are doing without changing your current habits. You can use any type of wearable device, a pedometer or an activity tracking device that can be found on your smartphone – your phone will already be recording your steps without you even knowing it! (Although you must keep the phone with you for that to work.) It really doesn't matter what you use, all that matters is that you find one you like and that you can afford, and you use it every day of the week.

Wearables that can measure water-based exercise or activities other than walking and running are great. This brings me to the biggest limitation with pedometers and accelerometers, as opposed to one you can wear around your wrist; you must clip it to your waist, which makes it easy to lose and not so practical to attach to certain clothing. It also won't allow you to measure activities such as cycling, rowing and swimming. Apple, Fitbit and Garmin market watches that are comprehensive devices you can use with all activities, but they come at a considerable cost to the consumer.

This first week of monitoring your current activity level will form part of your wash-out month, so that you can see how much you are currently moving before changing it. It's very common for my patients to think they are moving much more than they are, and this simple task will give you a true indication of your baseline level. Work out your average steps for the week and write it down. After you get an indication of your baseline level of exercise during the first week of the wash-out period, it's then time to address the fifth principle of the IWL plan – *Choose to move*. This means focusing on your incidental activity and not worrying about struc-tured activity just yet. It may take a few months to get to my suggested level of incidental physical activity (10,000 steps per day) and that is fine and advised. It's all about making gradual but real-istic and sustainable changes that become a way of life. The gradual increase in your incidental activity level – for example, by initially walking for 10 minutes per day and building up to 30 minutes per day over the course of a month – will also ensure you don't end up injuring yourself or exacerbating joint pain from the excess body weight you are carrying around. Start off by selecting one or two of the suggestions on this list that are practical for you. These will form some of the first positive habits during your wash-out month (from week two onwards, after you get an indication of your baseline activity level).

1. Use the stairs instead of the lift.

2. Take 10-minute breaks from your desk, at least three times per day.

3. Park further away from your workplace to incorporate walking to and from your car.

4. Get off one bus stop earlier than your usual stop.

5. Take public transport instead of driving.

5. Walk or cycle to the shops.

6. Take phone calls while walking around.

7. Use social catch-ups as an opportunity for exercise – instead of going to the coffee shop or the pub, meet your friends for a kick around, a swim or a stroll.

8. Park at the back of the car park to make you walk further to the shops or your workplace.

9. Trial a walking meeting. I love these and so do my colleagues!

If you are not currently performing any activity, the 10,000 steps per day (or equivalent movement in cycling or swimming – explained later in the chapter) should form part of your wash-out period (see Chapter 5). I appreciate that steps are not a good measure for everyone, because many people are unable to walk very far. If you are one of these people, it means turning your legs over on a stationary bike or getting in the pool to move around, and if you have an Apple watch, a Garmin or a Fitbit it will measure these activities. Even though you are embarking on the IWL plan from the get-go, remember that you may need to accept that a few months are often needed to wash out the previous dieting history and allow your weight to reset at its 'set point' (that is, if you're still regaining from a recent diet attempt). This also gives you ample time to get to an incidental activity level that becomes habitual and easy to incorporate into your daily routine. Sudden increases in activity are *not* advised, because you will only end up injured.

Incorporating structured activity

Once you have adjusted your way of life to focus more on opportune movement you can then start to work on what is needed to achieve the small amount of weight loss (approximately 0.5 kg) required per week on the IWL plan. This involves incorporating structured activity and, specifically, 30 minutes of moderate-intensity (I'll come back to this soon) activity, such as walking, cycling or swimming, five days per week. As you progress, you should also look to include some muscle-strengthening exercises that you can complete in the comfort of your own home.

Muscle-strengthening exercises might conjure up images of singlet-clad men grunting in the gym, but it's as easy as doing something in the comfort of your own home and you don't need weights. You can use objects from your house (such as food cans) and it's also enough to just do exercises using your body weight (such as squats and push-ups). You will find plenty of exercise programs on YouTube, which include 30-minute standing and seated resistance videos that anyone can do without the need for equipment, as well as through the Interval Weight Loss online program, available at intervalweightloss.com.au.

You certainly shouldn't embark on a strenuous exercise routine if you haven't exercised for a while. You are putting yourself at risk of potential heart attack and you need to start gradually with low- to moderate-intensity exercise. You're also likely to end up injured or with a very painful muscular side effect called delayed onset muscle soreness (DOMS). DOMS is nothing to worry about, but it's a very painful consequence of the muscle fibres breaking down, resulting in a lot of pain with even small movements. You will end up with DOMS if you haven't exercised in a while or if you try a new exercise. A health screen at your general practitioner/primary-care provider is also advised if you haven't done any exercise in six months or more.

I have worked with patients with different limitations – size, pain, mobility issues – but they all end up moving. Every stage of life presents an opportunity, so don't keep making excuses that you don't have time to move or you are in too much pain to move. This comes back to the identity excuses we discussed in Chapter 2. We are all busy in this modern time-poor environment. Block off some time in your calendar every day for structured exercise – the 30 minutes you do will add more than 30 minutes to your productivity. It's a net gain, which is even more relevant for those who are too busy to exercise.

Achieving the 30 minutes of activity can be broken up into blocks of 10 minutes if you're time poor, your mobility is limited, or your joints can't cope. The best type of exercise is walking, wading in the pool or cycling on a stationary bike when first starting out. Once you build up to include 30 minutes of structured activity five days per week, you can start to mix up your routine by including other activities such as swimming and some strength training, starting at one and building up to two days per week. This is particularly relevant during the weight-loss months.

Several of my patients have found that sleeping in their exercise gear gets them up and going first thing, with no time to make excuses. Yes, it seems crazy but it works for many. Another good option is wearing shoes appropriate to walking on your commute. For instance, you could get off the bus early and walk half an hour to your place of work, then put on your heels or dress shoes. You might not like how it looks, but I'm sure you'll like how you look when you're your new IWL self. You can also dance, paddleboard, garden, play tennis, or run – or jog! – around an oval with your kids.

What activity is best?

All activities are great. The most important thing is to participate in physical activities that you enjoy, to exercise with others and to explore different environments. Don't go to places you dislike or can't afford. Many of my patients join a gym, thinking that the expense of a membership will coax them into attending. Sadly, most of them find that two weeks after signing they stop going, though they continue to see money being deducted from their account.

Many people just don't want to go to the gym as it only intensifies their lack of self-worth because they're not as slim or fit or toned or strong as other people, and as a result they give up. Some people also find the hassle of going somewhere specific to do something they aren't especially keen on too much of a burden. The whole notion of getting in your car and driving somewhere to work out is absolute madness. If anything, you should be walking there! This is not to say you have to rule out the gym environment completely. But before you sign up, try a few different ones to ensure it is the one for you. They should offer a free trial and many even have a good peer-support network where you can discuss your challenges with like-minded people or find someone to train with. It doesn't matter if it's classes you are looking for, or areas to work out solo, or a dance class if you danced growing up; all that matters is that it's the right environment for you. This can be especially relevant if you have young ones because some have a childcare facility for when you work out.

Others simply prefer to walk, cycle or swim. Walking is particularly good post-pregnancy because you can walk the streets while pushing the pram. Not all exercise needs to be high intensity. There is certainly benefit in mixing up the type of exercise and intensity (I'll get to this soon), but the IWL plan has no interest in getting you to partake in activities that you don't like.

Why won't the weight budge?

When you first start on the IWL plan, it is important to have realistic expectations. Specifically, don't get disheartened if you don't see the weight decrease on the scales. Statistically speaking, you are likely to fall in that 70 per cent of the population that I just told you about, who don't meet the bare minimum of 30 minutes of exercise five days per week. But before you start to see the weight shift, what you will get is the many other physical and mental health benefits that are attributed to exercise. Even with just low levels of exercise you will experience a decrease in depressive symptoms, an improvement in mood and vitality, and a reduced chance of developing disease, such as type 2 diabetes and cardiovascular disease.

Exercise will help you lose weight once you get to a manageable and sustainable volume. And importantly, it will result in an improvement in your body composition and prevent muscle decline. Our muscle mass naturally declines at around age 40, and this decline accelerates at age 50 – a process known as sarcopenia. Exercise actively protects and builds up your muscle mass and prevents this process from occurring. It will also prevent the weight gain that many attribute to menopause or a slowing metabolism with age. This is because muscle is much more metabolically active than fat, meaning it burns more energy at rest and prevents your metabolism from decreasing. In fact, the amount your metabolism decreases with age is minute (unless you have spent a lifetime dieting); the main reason it does is through a lack of exercise. Hence, the overall goal with weight loss on the IWL plan is to maintain as much of your muscle mass as possible and to see the weight loss coming predominantly from fat stores. Simply put, the more muscle mass you have, the more calories you will burn.

Exercise as a medicine

You need to view exercise as a medicine. Physical activity activates the brain's pleasure circuit. Just like cigarettes, alcohol, drugs or food, exercise too can become an addiction. Exercise will boost your serotonin levels, consequently improving your mood and social functioning and help you make healthier food choices. Better still, it will help prevent impulsive food choices and is one of the best forms of stress management. What I am telling you is that if you can get your exercise routine into gear, everything else will fall into place. You will learn to love exercise and look forward to it each day because it will become your medicine and your new addiction. Exercise needn't follow strict routines, anything that gets you moving is just fine.

How much exercise is safe during pregnancy?

Safe levels of exercise vary for pregnant women and it is always important to consult with your doctor before commencing any exercise program, particularly during pregnancy. They will screen you to assess your level of risk, as it is dangerous for anyone to jump straight into an exercise program if they have been doing very little.

You should be incorporating at least 30 minutes of moderate-intensity exercise five days per week and, wherever possible, two days of strength-training exercises that can be completed in the comfort of your own home. (Some body-weight strengthening exercises are provided in this chapter.) Of course, you can do more than this, but remember you're growing a person during pregnancy, so it's not a time to reach new fitness heights. Instead, your goal should be to maintain your exercise level as per the weight-maintenance months of the IWL plan (more on this later), particularly during the latter stages of pregnancy when you may start to feel a little more uncomfortable. This is a time to continue with your exercise routine but with a focus on reduced intensity and avoiding the introduction of new activities.

Importantly, regular exercise throughout pregnancy will help you carry the weight you gain, reduce complications associated with pregnancy (such as carrying a large baby, miscarriage and stillbirth), prepare you for the physical challenge of labour and birth, improve your mood and vitality, improve your sleep quality, and help you bounce back quicker to your pre-pregnancy weight following the delivery of your child.

Which exercises are best during pregnancy?

The best type of exercise is one that gets you moving and that you enjoy, without causing physical distress. Your focus should be on including plenty of aerobic exercise such as walking, running, swimming, cycling, aqua aerobics, yoga, Pilates and specific pregnancy exercise classes that your gym may offer. If your gym doesn't offer pregnancy-specific classes, ensure you tell the instructor of any class you attend so they can modify according to your needs.

Building activity into your daily life is also vital; gardening, housework, walking between meetings and using the stairs instead of the lift are all important ways of increasing your incidental activity.

The pelvic floor

The pelvic floor is a group of muscles that support the organs (bladder, uterus and bowel) in your pelvis. It runs from the front of your pubic bone to your sitting bone at the back. If it's weak, gaps start to appear and parts of your bladder or bowel might start descending through them resulting in a leaky bladder or incontinence. The extra weight and force during pregnancy can weaken it.

Specific pelvic-floor stability exercises should be included every day, because a weak pelvic floor can result in all sorts of barriers to exercise. It can be hard to identify the right muscles; the easiest way to test is when sitting on the toilet for a wee. While midstream, stop the flow and hold for a few seconds – these are the muscles you are targeting. An easy and simple exercise to do every day is the pelvic squeeze. There are two variations of the same exercise that you should do three times a day. While standing, squeeze and lift the muscles as if you're trying to stop a wee. Hold the squeeze for up to five seconds and then relax for five seconds. Repeat 10 times (it will take you less than two minutes to complete). Build up to 10-second holds as your pelvic-floor strength increases. Following this, do three sets of 10 quick squeezes, without the five-second hold (each set will take approximately 10 seconds to complete, so three sets with a 10-second break in between will take you only a minute to complete). The great thing about this exercise is you can do it anywhere – for example, while waiting in the queue for the bus, waiting for your morning coffee, waiting at home for the kettle to boil, or talking to your colleague at work; no one will even know you're doing it.

At what intensity should you exercise during pregnancy?

The 'talk test' is a good guide to the intensity at which you should exercise. Focus on longer-duration activities where you can still maintain a conversation during the exercise. You can include high-intensity training, but you will find as your body changes during pregnancy so does your ability to exercise at higher intensities. This is particularly relevant beyond 16 weeks and this is the time to modify your training.

Are there any exercises to avoid during pregnancy?

You shouldn't be scared to exercise during pregnancy, but you need to take some precautions. First, you should stop exercising if you experience any pain, dizziness, light-headedness, weakness, blurred vision, excessive fatigue, shortness of breath before exertion or vaginal bleeding.

You should avoid all contact sports, scuba diving and any activities at high altitude (for example, skiing) during pregnancy. It's also not advised to partake in activities with an increased risk of falling, such trampolining, gymnastics and horse riding.

You can still lift weights, but you should focus on less resistance with higher repetitions, rather than heavy weights at low repetitions. Beyond 16 weeks' gestation it is best to perform exercises while standing, sitting or lying on your side. Exercising on your back can make you feel light-headed.

When is it safe to return to exercise after pregnancy?

Exercise will help you recover after childbirth, improve your mood, help prevent postnatal depression and strengthen your muscles.

There's plenty you can do to get your body moving but how soon after giving birth you can start moving will depend on your individual circumstances. It will also depend on how active you were before you had the baby and what sort of delivery (vaginal or caesarean) you had.

After a vaginal birth, you can start with gentle walking as soon as you feel up to it. Build up gradually until you can walk for 30 minutes. You should also recommence (you can do this straightaway) the variations of the pelvic-squeeze activity I previously described. Just as your body goes through big changes with pregnancy, it needs adequate time to recover. Therefore, you shouldn't do any strenuous activity for the first three months and you should wait until your postnatal check-up (typically six weeks after the birth) until you recommence swimming. A caesarean will require much more recovery time. But don't panic – the weight will still fall off you; you just need to let your body recover first. If you had a caesarean, you can recommence the pelvic-stability exercise straight after birth, but you should wait until your postnatal check-up until you recommence your exercise routine and you should start with light-impact activities such as walking or bike riding. Pushing your little one around the neighbourhood is a great place to start.

Exercising while breastfeeding

Breastfeeding can make it a little challenging to exercise, not only due to exhaustion from the regular feeding program throughout the night, but also due to some side effects that you may experience from breastfeeding itself (for example, tender breasts and sore, cracked nipples). Many of my patients talk of the struggles when it comes to fatigue after their baby is born, and often the last thing they want to do is run around the park. But, despite how tired you feel you must still prioritise exercise, because you will feel more energetic for doing it; it will help you not only physically but also mentally. Some of the most practical workouts involve simply pushing the pram around the neighbourhood and incorporating hills. When it comes to the best time to do it, this is between feeds, preferably straight after a feed to reduce the weight of your breasts (as they do fill up between feeds) and to avoid your baby becoming unsettled while you're out. It's also a good idea to provide extra protection for your nipples because the added friction from salty sweat running over sore and cracked nipples can be enough to deter you from vigorous exercise altogether.

Exercising with the kids around

This is another wonderful and opportune time to move. Kids love activity and you should use this to your advantage to move with them. Some of my most successful patients have had multiple children. Before I met them, they thought of entertaining the kids as a chore, but after realising the potential that all their energy offered, they too started to leverage off it. There is no reason you can't move when they move. If they want to play on the equipment, play with them. If they want to kick the ball, kick it with them. If they're playing sport, walk around the oval while watching. Your focus should simply be getting involved with them. And if that's not appropriate because they're playing with their friends, you can still exercise within eye view.

Some other great ways to increase your exercise with the kids is to walk them to school, go for family walks after dinner or ride your bikes instead of driving to the shops. If you find you're playing taxi driver all day, it might not always be practical to walk around the oval or do some other exercise while your kid is playing sport.

Of course, this would be the ideal situation, but if you're finding that you're dropping Charlotte at one event, Sally at the next and then Eddie 15 kilometres in the other direction, it's not practical to be active while they are. You'll find yourself sitting in the car the whole time. You might be able to team up with another parent and share the pick-ups and drop-offs or you might find that you can do a little movement at each drop-off. All those five-minute bursts of activity will add up. Otherwise, you will need to get up earlier in the morning and do it before you leave, schedule some alone time in the afternoon or take the kids out to play later in the day. There is always a way to incorporate exercise into your day and the kids will love it because there is nothing more they want to do than play.

Exercise and your menstrual cycle

Your menstrual cycle has a massive impact on your mood, metabolism, diet, strength, training and recovery. 'That time of the month' remains a taboo topic when it comes to physical activity, training and sport, but it's something that needs to be better understood so you optimise your success on the IWL plan. There is a physiological reason why some days you just don't feel like training at higher intensities and other days you feel ready to train like Rocky Balboa. In fact, the rise and fall of a woman's hormones during the 28-day cycle has a profound effect on exercise and performance as well as a range of other things within the body. The simplest way to monitor this is by using a smartphone app to track your menstrual cycle. This is the first step that will then allow you to sync your training schedule with your menstrual cycle.

Your hormones

Hormones are the chemical messengers that constantly carry important information about our bodies. For men, while their hormones change during their lifetime, day-to-day they remain pretty stable. On the other hand, for women, levels of sex hormones fluctuate daily with two hormone phases every month – high and low. Your cycle can be broken up into stages. Day 0–14 is known as the follicular phase. This includes the menstrual phase (first day of your period) to 14 days later. Your oestrogen levels increase during this phase and your progesterone stays stable.

During the low phase – the follicular phase – females are physiologically similar to males in metabolism and recovery. The low-hormone phase occurs in the first two weeks of the cycle (the arrival of your period marks day one of week one). This is the time to train hard; the time to focus on higher intensity exercise and a large variety of exercise, especially if in a weight-loss month on the IWL plan. You will feel less pain and recover faster; training will feel easier. And you will start to feel even more energetic towards the end of the two-week follicular phase. One week into your cycle is when your metabolic rate is at its lowest point, so it's another good reason to make the most of working out hard during this phase to help offset metabolic slow-down. At approximately day 12 of your menstrual cycle, your oestrogen level surges, as does the level of luteinising hormone, triggering ovulation. You will feel strongest and most energetic at this point, allowing you to work-out harder and focus better on your goals. You may also start to feel hungrier as your metabolism picks back up again.

During the second half of the cycle, the high-hormone phase – the luteal phase – progesterone levels peak, resulting in decreases in strength, aerobic capacity and ability to tolerate heat. When you are in this phase, exercising can feel like an uphill struggle and you will fatigue quicker. Your body burns more fat during this phase as the change in hormones makes it harder for you to access glycogen (carbohydrate) stores. So, this is the time to incorporate lower intensity cardio, low-intensity strength training, active recovery sessions such as an easy swim, yoga and stretching, and walking. High progesterone increases the amount of salt you lose from the body, delays sweat response and raises your core temperature by about 0.5 degree Celsius, making you prone to heat stress and more easily fatigued during workouts. It also breaks down muscle so you won't enjoy the same gains from your workouts and recovery is slower. And coupled with all of this, fluid shifts from your blood plasma to your cells, causing you to feel bloated, thickening your blood and raising your blood pressure, and making you more predisposed to central nervous system fatigue – simply put, exercise feels harder than usual. The level of the sleep hormone melatonin rises during the luteal phase, so you crave more rest. Your metabolism does increase by 5–10 per cent during this phase, so your appetite increases too, and by about 1250 kilojoules per day. But, the best way to manage all of this is still exercise, just of the low-intensity variety. And make sure to drink plenty of water, too.

It seems counter-intuitive but when your period starts, you will start to feel normal again. Hormone levels return to baseline and you will be able to start including some more high-intensity training. However, everyone is different and you need to work out what works best for you.

By recognising these phases of your menstrual cycle, you will know how to deal with common symptoms of tiredness, irritability, fluid retention and headaches, and not be discouraged along the way. A well-planned exercise program will allow you to work with your cycle, not against it. It will also allow you to see better results.

Ella, an IWL community member, became very disheartened a few months into the IWL program. A couple of months after starting her new way of life she re-found her love for exercise after being sedentary for nearly a decade. A local gym offered a range of structured classes that she loved, including boxing, bike and a weights circuit – all high-intensity stuff. After all the classes she would be knackered but also energetic and pumped for the day ahead. Some weeks she would feel energetic and find the classes tough but manageable. Then there were days when she could barely get herself out of bed and would go to the class feeling tired, weak and less able to perform at her desired intensity. In fact, some of the sessions she would even leave early, disappointed with her effort. I saw that all of Ella's training was hard. Whenever she exercised, she put in 100 per cent, which is great but not always practical and certainly not always necessary. After teaching her more about how the body works and the typical 28-days of a menstrual cycle, she felt relieved knowing that this was normal and that others were also going through the same issues. She hadn't noticed it in the past because she hadn't been incorporating high-intensity exercise into her weekly exercise plan. In fact, she hadn't been performing any structured activity at all. We made some simple switches to her activity routine so that each month would include a mix of high-intensity training during the two weeks of the follicular phase, and then more lower-intensity and active recovery sessions like yoga during the luteal phase of her cycle. She also didn't worry about the number on the scales when she was retaining fluid and feeling bloated, just before her period. She knew the number would correct itself at the next weigh-in. This change in her activity plan allowed her to achieve her goals during the IWL weight-loss months, and it also meant she was much happier knowing that she now had better control over her body and that she needed to work with it, rather than against it.

How much exercise do you need to do to lose weight?

As you have just learnt, your first goal is to build up your incidental activity and slowly incorporate more structured activity so you can reach the 30 minutes of moderate-intensity exercise most days of the week (this includes two strength-training days). You need to work towards 10,000 steps per day, which is the level that you should be able to sustain every day of the week. And remember, it doesn't have to be walking, it can be swimming, cycling or housework instead. As with your body weight, your daily steps should also be written down so you can track your progress each week. Even though your Apple watch, Fitbit or Garmin will store your data, you need to visualise it on a graph. Some days will be a little less and others will be a little more. It's the average that you are monitoring, and if you can reach an average of 10,000 steps per day over the course of the week, this will ensure you are looking after your health. However, depending on your dieting history and your current weight, this may not be enough to help you lose weight (larger people will lose weight more easily, as will those who haven't dieted before). It will also depend on what activities and intensities you have worked at to get to your 10,000 steps per day. If it was all high-intensity sprints on the grass, for example, and involved a lot of moderate and vigorous-intensity activities resulting in you sweating most of the day, it's more than likely plenty. On the contrary, if your 10,000 steps per day were largely made up of light-intensity strolls, it's unlikely you will see yourself losing weight. Ultimately, you want to see the 10,000 steps as ancillary to your structured exercise. And remember, steps is just an inter-changeable term for movement. If you are achieving the equivalent of 10,000 steps on a stationary bike this is also fine and likely to see you losing weight if you are getting up a sweat and your heart rate is high. Use the rough guide of 20 minutes on the bike being equivalent to about 3000 steps. For a lot of people, it's usually the addition of a small amount of structured activity such as a social game of soccer or a gym class on top of the 10,000 steps per day, or a change in the type of activity you are doing that will get you into a weight-loss phase.

You need to establish what works for you, and some people are more time-poor than others. For example, Jane, a current member of the IWL community, is a full-time investment banker and a single mother of two children. After dropping off the kids each day at school, she often gets stuck at work later than she hoped and has to pick them up from after-school care. She is extremely time-poor but since learning about the IWL plan has made the switch to prioritise her health. On the days she takes the kids to after-school sport, she works out at the same time – keeping an eye on them but still exercising at the same park. On the days this is not possible and she is likely to work late, she will block off time in her calendar to ensure that every lunchtime she makes time to go outdoors. Sometimes it's the gym, sometimes the oval, and other times just a walk. She also monitors her steps on her smartphone and ensures she hits the 10,000 steps per day through incidental movement at work.

How do you know what intensity to work at?

The sweat factor is one of the best guides, even for those who don't typically sweat. Increasing your walking speed is a straightforward way to increase the intensity. When I refer to moderate-intensity exercise, this is where you are walking at a pace that makes you huff and puff and sweat. It's not practical for everyone to start at this intensity but this is what I want you to work towards. For those who struggle to do 30 minutes in one go, that's fine, because research has shown that if you break your physical activity up into two shorter bouts per day this can be more effective for weight loss than physical activity undertaken in a single long bout (for example, 2 × 20-minute walks, instead of 1 × 40-minute walk each day). This is because you're more likely and able to work out harder if the duration is shorter.

Put simply, if you are sweating, you are doing it right. This is particularly relevant if you are achieving your 10,000 steps per day, or equivalent movement from cycling or swimming, pre-dominantly from structured rather than incidental activity. In this instance you are probably relying on structured activity to achieve your goal and are likely to be very sedentary in your day-to-day life. The problem here is, if you don't keep up the structured activity, you will find you are barely moving at all. This is often seen in people who adopt the all-or-nothing approach. This approach is not healthy, not sustainable and not advised. As per the goal of the wash-out month, you should first work out how you can increase your movement without the reliance on structured activity – after all, it's not always practical to take a few hours out of your day for structured activity time.

Increase in appetite with exercise

Many people report an increase in hunger following exercise. Despite what the research shows (that this is not usually the case), you need to listen to your body and give it the nutrition it requires. All the same principles of the IWL plan still apply. You should never deprive yourself of food and if you feel hungry, you should eat, but always remember to *reach for nature first*. Think of an increase in hunger as your body telling you it is starting to work more efficiently and that it is responding to the new stresses (physical activity) you have introduced. Embrace it, don't fear it!

Preventing injury and setbacks

The goal of the IWL plan is to get you moving and it truly doesn't matter what form of exercise you do as long as you adopt a sensible approach that doesn't see you with DOMS, injured or with aching joints that restrict your movement. This only ends up in disappointment, and it will happen if you do too much too soon. It will not only set you back with respect to your physical goals on the IWL plan, but it will also influence your mental health. Not being able to exercise can result in frustration but also because of your newfound addiction for exercise, you will become dependent on the high you get from those feel-good chemicals triggered in the brain while exercising.

It is vital to start off gradually while keeping the long-term goal at the front of your mind. The excess body weight you are carrying will impose undue stress on your joints, which is exacerbated when taking part in certain exercise and this includes walking. You must gradually increase the amount of exercise you do, just like an athlete would gradually increase the amount of training they do. Drastic changes in activity or intensity are not advised.

Depending on your current body weight, this may mean solely participating in non-body weight bearing exercise to alleviate the stress off your joints. For others, it may also mean starting off and performing exercise while seated. Joint pain is a common complaint for a large percentage of the population. In this instance, most incidental exercise will not be practical and you will only be able to achieve the recommended amount of physical activity through the incorporation of non-body weight bearing exercise such as swimming, cycling and rowing. Aiming to include cycling in small, frequent bouts on a stationary bike in the convenience of your own home can be particularly beneficial if you're too self-conscious to exercise in public. Recumbent bikes are good because the seats are comfortable, allowing you to exercise for long periods of time without the common complaint of a sore saddle post-riding. Swimming is another great exercise that takes the stress off your joints, as is completing a seated gym routine with tins of food as the resistance. It doesn't matter what you do on the bike, in the pool, or in your home gym environment, all that matters is that you move.

The great thing about exercising in the pool is that many of the activity-monitoring devices these days are waterproof and allow you to track your activity whatever the environment. If you are using a pedometer or similar device that you can't take in the pool, the general rule of thumb is that every 20 minutes of moderate activity equates to approximately 3000 steps. Once your weight starts to drop and you alleviate some of the pain and stress off your joints, you will find that walking becomes easier and you will gradually be able to increase your activity by incorporating more incidental exercise – a crucial step on your weight-loss journey.

For those who can perform body weight bearing exercise, you must start off by incorporating a day of non-body weight bearing exercise in between each day. For example, walk Monday (body weight bearing), bike Tuesday (non-body weight bearing), walk Wednesday (body weight bearing), swim Thursday (non-body weight bearing), gym Friday (body weight bearing), row machine Saturday (non-body weight bearing), and so on. This will give your muscles and joints time to recover between exercise sessions. Otherwise, you too will end up with an injury.

Appropriate clothing for exercise

It's challenging enough finding the courage to get moving, especially if you feel like everyone is gazing at you every time you walk out the door. It can be even harder to find appropriate and supportive clothing for your body shape and size. However, this is important because without it, you're less likely to enjoy exercise and more likely to hurt yourself. Shop for breathable and comfortable clothing that you feel good in. If you're shopping online, choose a site that offers free returns and exchanges, because you almost certainly won't get it right the first time.

One of the biggest problem areas for women is their breasts. Big or small, everyone has them. However, one in five women report that their breasts stop them from exercising, with size, self-consciousness and pain reported as the most common barriers to physical activity.

It's crucial to find a sports bra that's the correct size. Simply using a tape measure isn't going to cut it, nor is an everyday bra for sport. There are professional bra-fitting criteria that are important to use. Many of my patients have also benefitted from wearing two bras and wearing a sports top with built-in breast support panels.

Swimming can be another challenge. A swimming costume alone is not enough to protect big breasts, so it's important to track one down with moulded cups and adjustable straps to give more support.

Continuous versus high-intensity interval training

High-intensity interval training, popularly known as HIIT training, has become a hot topic of late. And no wonder. After all, who wouldn't want to get the same benefits (burn fat and get fit) from exercise but in a quarter or half the time it usually takes? The main reason people say they don't exercise is a perceived lack of time. For those unfamiliar with the concept of HIIT training, it involves incorporating bouts of very high intensity (i.e. working at high heart rates) for short periods of time, followed by periods of low intensity to recover, before repeating, and so on, until you complete the prescribed session. For example, you would peddle as hard as you can on a stationary bike (a recumbent bike is perfectly fine) for 10 seconds (the 'on' period), before then easing off and peddling easy for 30 seconds so you can get your breath back (the 'off' period). You keep repeating this 'on' and 'off' period, exercising the whole time, until 15 or 20 minutes is up. This is just one example. Another example might be while walking. You could walk fast for one minute and then walk at a slower pace while getting your breath back for two minutes, repeating until you have walked for a set amount of time (again, it might be 10 or 20 minutes). The theory is that you can burn just as many calories and therefore just as much fat in half the amount of time as aerobic exercise (for example, a long slow walk for 40 minutes). Not because you burn more energy during the exercise (in fact, you will burn less energy as you switch to predominantly using carbohydrate as opposed to fat as a fuel source when the intensity of exercise increases), but because you burn more energy at rest (post-exercise). This is due to a term known as exercise post oxygen consumption (EPOC) following exercise. With HIIT training (which is considered a form of vigorous physical activity), there is a lack of oxygen available during exercise, resulting in more oxygen being required post-exercise to recuperate (which consequently burns more energy). HIIT is a great thing to include in your exercise plan on the IWL plan, but there is a catch. For the younger population (those aged around 20) in a healthy BMI range (23 kg/m²), HIIT training works just as well as continuous exercise for fat loss and improving fitness level, because this group of people can get their heart rate up and push themselves to work at the harder intensities. But for many of us, due to a large amount of excess body weight, it is very hard to get to the required intensities during the 'on' bouts where you need to work as hard as you can for the set amount of time. Despite this, even though you won't burn as many calories during a HIIT session as you would in a continuous aerobic session, HIIT sessions are a wonderful addition to your repertoire of physical activities that you can add to your weekly plan, especially on days when you are time poor. And it doesn't matter what size you are, anyone can do them. The session I just described on a recumbent bike is one such example. Plus, it adds the necessary variety that you need to 'shock' the body. You will also find that once you start to lose some weight, you will better tolerate the higher-intensity sessions. I strongly encourage you to include a version (any of your own versions are fine) of a HIIT session into your IWL plan. You can use the following program as an example of how to gradually increase your training over a 12-week period. It is important to start gradually, and slowly build up. The same applies for continuous exercise. Start with 10–15 minutes and over time you will be able to build up to 30–45-minute walks with no trouble at all. You can do these sessions on a bike, while walking or running, or in the pool. Each session should be accompanied by a 6-minute warm-up at a low intensity/resistance.

Week 1: 30 seconds 'on', 180 seconds 'off', repeat 4 times. Including warm-up and cool-down this will total 20 minutes. (NB: The cool-down for each session is the last 'off' component.)

Week 2: 30 seconds on, 180 seconds off, repeat 4 times. Including warm-up and cool-down this will total 20 minutes.

Week 3: 30 seconds on, 180 seconds off, repeat 5 times. Including warm-up and cool-down this will total 23:30 minutes.

Week 4: 30 seconds on, 180 seconds off, repeat 5 times. Including warm-up and cool-down this will total 23:30 minutes.

Week 5: 30 seconds on, 120 seconds off, repeat 6 times. Including warm-up and cool-down this will total 21 minutes.

Week 6: 30 seconds on, 120 seconds off, repeat 6 times. Including warm-up and cool-down this will total 21 minutes.

Week 7: 45 seconds on, 120 seconds off, repeat 6 times. Including warm-up and cool-down this will total 22:30 minutes.

Week 8: 45 seconds on, 120 seconds off, repeat 6 times. Including warm-up and cool-down this will total 22:30 minutes.

Week 9: 60 seconds on, 180 seconds off, repeat 5 times. Including warm-up and cool-down this will total 26 minutes.

Week 10: 60 seconds on, 180 seconds off, repeat 5 times. Including warm-up and cool-down this will total 26 minutes.

Week 11: 60 seconds on, 120 seconds off, repeat 6 times. Including warm-up and cool-down this will total 24 minutes.

Week 12: 60 seconds on, 120 seconds off, repeat 6 times. Including warm-up and cool-down this will total 24 minutes.

Exercise during the weight-loss months

During the weight-loss months of the IWL plan it is important to continually change your exercise routine. This means trying new walking or running routes, working at higher intensities by incorporating hills or trialling new exercises or activities you have not done before (for example, at the gym or alternative sports). The higher intensities can be performed on any equipment – bike, rower or in the pool (this is where HIIT sessions come in).

The variety of activity during the weight-loss months should not be confined to the type of exercise alone. It also applies to where you are exercising. I'm referring to the physical location itself – the streets you are walking on, the ovals you are training at and the people you are exercising with. Every time you exercise somewhere different you gain a new energy that you didn't know existed – not only the location but also the excitement of going somewhere new. Every location offers something that the previous place didn't and this is the stimulus that you need to stay motivated and, importantly, to achieve the results you are after. And never disregard the importance of incidental activity – everyday life offers us multiple opportunities to get fit, if we choose to take them.

Following is an example week of exercise during the weight-loss months.

Monday: Spin class before work (if you normally go to yoga, go to spin instead to switch it up!). *NB: This is a non-body weight bearing exercise day.*

Tuesday: 30-minute walk incorporating hills to make it a HIIT session. You can do this while pushing the pram or you could do a fast shuffle/jog around the oval with a walk lap recovery while your child is playing sport. This would also be a form of HIIT, because the fast shuffle/jog will be at a higher intensity than the walk recovery.

Wednesday: 1-hour cycle to and from work or a 1-hour cycle around the neighbourhood with your little one strapped to the back. *NB: This is a non-body weight bearing exercise day.*

Thursday: Gym class while your toddler is in childcare.

Friday: At home bodyweights workout while seated – see examples that follow (you can also find hundreds of these on YouTube). *NB: This is a non-body weight bearing exercise day.*

Saturday: Game of soccer with the kids; walk to and from a new coffee shop in the neighbouring suburbs; or walk to the supermarket and carry your groceries home.

Sunday: Swimming at aqua aerobics session. *NB: This is a non-body weight bearing exercise day.*

Example bodyweight workouts you can do in the comfort of your own home

Complete each of the listed exercises as a circuit and complete three circuits in total with a break of 3–5 minutes in between each set. If you can't complete the recommended time and reps listed, don't worry, it's a goal you can gradually work towards and then surpass. You can use resistance bands or even cans of food for extra resistance. These exercises can be done anywhere and cost nothing.

Session 1

1. Plank: In a push-up position with legs and body straight, focus on your core while distributing weight evenly across forearms, elbows and toes. Hold for 30 seconds.

2. Walking lunges: Stay upright and walk forward with each lunge, making sure your front knee does not bend past your toes, and your back leg should touch the ground. Complete 10 each leg.

3. Knee push-ups: A great way to start off before heading into the full push-up position. Ensure your back is flat and lower yourself by bending at the elbows to where your chest touches the ground and push back up in a slow controlled fashion. Complete 12 reps.

4. Side plank: Begin in the plank position and then roll your body to the side, lifting your arm overhead. Stack your feet and lift through the hip to keep a nice straight line. Return to your plank position before repeating on the other side. Hold for 20 seconds each side.

5. Squats: Start upright and lower gradually until you mimic sitting in a chair, before then pushing back up with your legs while keeping your back straight. Complete 20 reps.

6. Hundreds: Lie on your back with your knees bent and up in the air, forming a 90-degree angle. Lift forward into a crunch position and pulse your arms for 100 beats.

7. Walk sit: Move into the squat position with knees and thighs at 90 degrees and walk gradually forward, taking small steps to maintain a squat position. Walk for 30 seconds.

Session 2

1. Standing lunges: Stay upright and step forward with one leg (making sure your front knee does not bend past your toes, and your back leg should touch the ground), and push back to standing position. Complete 15 each leg.

2. Tricep dips: Using a bench seat, step or something similar, place your hands behind you with your fingers pointing in the same direction as your feet. Lower your body by bending at the elbows and then push back up by pressing and straightening your elbows until your arms are fully extended. Complete 20 reps.

3. Ice skaters: Sit in a squat position and slide your foot behind you across the body as if you are mimicking an ice-skating movement. Complete 20 each side.

4. Mountain climbers: In a plank position, draw your knee across the body to your opposite elbow. Complete 50 reps.

5. Bear crawls: On your hands and toes, knees off the ground, crawl up and down the lounge room. Crawl for 30 seconds.

6. Calf raises: Stand upright on a step with your heels hanging off the back, push up to your toes and lower until your heels fall just below the step level. Complete 20 reps.

7. Shoulder taps while in plank position on hands and toes: Pick up one hand at a time and tap the opposite shoulder by pulling your arm over your body. Complete 12 each side.

Session 3

1. Star jumps: In a standing position extend the limbs and attain maximum height while focusing on power throughout the mid-section. Complete 40 jumps.

2. Toe touches: In a crunch position with legs straight up in the air, reach up and touch toes. Complete 30 touches.

3. Running on spot: Run on the spot and pump your legs up and down as fast as you can. Run for 30 seconds.

4. Russian twists: Sit with legs bent in the air at 90 degrees, rotate your body from side to side with arms out in front of you. Complete 20 each side.

5. Chair squats: Sit in a squat position with knees at 90 degrees. Hold for 30 seconds.

6. Oblique side bend: Stand upright and drop one arm down your body as far as you can, while bending only at the waist. Complete 20 each side.

7. Half burpees: Stand tall and bend your knees and lower hips while placing your hands to the outside of your feet. Kick your legs back until they are straight, to mimic a push-up position, and reverse movement back to start. Complete 20 reps.

NB: If you are unsure how to do any of the above exercises, you can watch how to do each one at the Interval Weight Loss website.

Measuring your progress

Some of the best success stories on the IWL plan are told by people who track their improvements in fitness and strength along the way. There's an old saying: 'What gets measured, gets managed.' Seeing an improvement in your score is motivating. It could be as simple as having one activity that you perform at regular time periods (each month) to monitor your progress. For example, the time it takes you to swim 500 metres in the pool, the time it takes you to row 1 kilometre on the machine at the gym, the number of push-ups you can do in 30 seconds or the amount of weight you can put on the bar for squats. It doesn't matter what it is, they all provide a good benchmark that you can measure your progress against – progress breeds progress.

Exercise during the weight-maintenance months

The great thing is that the weight-maintenance months (every second month) allow you to ease off with the intensity, to forget about the variety and to be less diligent. This is a time to give your body a rest. You don't need to sweat it out during the weight-maintenance months, you just need to keep moving. During the weight-maintenance months, your 10,000 steps per day with light activities can be your exercise – depending on how much you wish to increase your consumption of treat foods or takeaway foods during these months. This will be a little trial-and-error when you first start; remember, what you are looking for is the trend in weight change over time. And for the weight-maintenance months you want that trend to stay relatively flat.

Tasks

Task 1

Using your phone or wearable device, start measuring your current activity level (particularly focusing on your incidental activity). During the first week of your wash-out month, don't change your current activity level, because you need an accurate baseline measure of how many steps per day you are doing. You can then use this as a baseline measure of your current activity level and start to increase it – gradually! If you don't have a wearable device, it is well worth the investment.

Task 2

The second thing you need to do is add structured activity to your calendar (a month's worth) with non-body weight bearing exercise between days of body weight bearing exercise. You don't have to include structured exercise every day (perhaps every second day to start) but you need to gradually build it up over the month.

CHAPTER 11

THE SIXTH PRINCIPLE: NO BLUE LIGHT AFTER TWILIGHT

Sleep is another vital piece of the puzzle towards success on the IWL plan. Research has shown that a loss of sleep results in risk taking and when it comes to food, this means poor meal choices. When we subject people to sleep deprivation in the lab – anything less than seven hours of sleep – it reduces the responsiveness of the brain to planning, reasoning and the future. On the contrary, we see a heightened responsiveness of the brain when it comes to food reward. What I'm saying is, you're more likely to reach for that chocolate bar when you're sleep deprived. And this can be extremely challenging during pregnancy, with a newborn or when juggling kids with disrupted sleep patterns.

Implementing each of the principles of the IWL plan to date will go a long way towards improving your sleep quality, but the sixth principle – *No blue light after twilight* – also plays a vital role. You must aim to get seven to eight hours of sleep per night. Yes, I can hear your responses: 'I don't have time for that!' 'I've never been able to sleep.' 'I only get four hours' sleep a night.' 'My partner keeps me awake with his snoring.' These are more identity excuses that you need to turn into identity-accountability statements to take ownership of your health. It may just be more rest that you need and by getting into bed at the same time each night and waking at the same time each morning, you will give your body the best chance of getting the rest it needs. In fact, recent research suggests that a regular bedtime and wake-up schedule is vital for weight management. When it comes to snoring, if you or your partner snore, see your doctor. Weight loss will help with this but there are also effective treatments for snoring (usually due to a condition known as sleep apnoea), which might be needed to improve your sleep quality until you lose weight. Even if you must sleep in separate rooms for a short period of time!

Pregnancy and sleep

When it comes to pregnancy and sleep, women can experience many issues. A common grievance is insomnia. Many women struggle to fall asleep or stay asleep due to stress and anxiety about labour and motherhood, as well as discomfort due to lower back pain, breast pain, pelvic girdle pain, nausea and baby movements. Other problems include reflux (heartburn), restless legs (unpleasant feeling in the legs), sleep apnoea (interrupted breathing during sleep) and frequent night-time urination. However, you can manage most of these challenges with the following tips.

1. Exercise every day.

2. Read or write in bed instead of forcing yourself to sleep.

3. Take a warm bath before bed.

4. Avoid too much spicy or fried food.

5. Ask your doctor about potential medication use for heartburn.

6. If snoring has become a habit, let your doctor know so they can determine whether you should be screened for sleep apnoea.

7. Drink most of your fluid intake at the start of the day and taper off from 4pm onwards.

8. Add a dimmer switch or night-light to the bathroom to avoid having to turn on the light each time you wake during the night.

Newborns and sleep deprivation

Sleep deprivation is no joke for new mums. Just when you manage to get on top of all the sleep issues caused during pregnancy, new problems can arise after you give birth. Each mum will experience different challenges but the most common relate to frequency of the feeding schedule, difficulties getting your baby to fall asleep and developmental challenges such as teething and growth spurts. Before allowing your sleep deprivation to hit rock bottom you should implement the following tips.

1. Change your routine. You may think that turning on the TV after your little one goes to sleep is your time to unwind and relax but it's going to do more harm than good. Not only will it increase your chance of comfort eating, it will also see you getting less rest. You need to adjust your sleep routine after your baby is born and ensure you go to bed at the same time each night and much earlier than you are used to.

2. Seek professional help and implement sleep training if you think it will be beneficial. There are various methods and I'm not here to add to the collection of sleep-training books,

but it's something you might consider, possibly when your baby is as young as four months.

3. Sleep when your baby sleeps. There is no harm in lying down when your baby does. A short nap can be all that's needed and those 20-minute naps quickly add up.

4. Lean on friends and family for assistance if you're able to. Often your parents or in-laws are more than happy to help and it might give you that little bit of help you need to ensure extra rest.

5. Consider pumping. If you have a partner or someone who can help, pump some breastmilk ahead of time, so they can take control of one of the feeding shifts.

The three most important things

Sleep is a big challenge for all women, irrespective of whether you are pregnant or have children. Workplace stressors are a common complaint and there are three things that everyone needs to implement when it comes to improving sleep quality.

The first one relates to technology. The modern-day environment has seen us develop a great fondness for technology and screens, which brings us to the sixth principle of the IWL plan – *No blue light after twilight*. This means removing all technology from the bedroom, and yes, that includes the television along with computers and phones. It should be a place of sanctuary, not work. And this applies to your children's rooms as well. Don't use any form of device before going to sleep and keep them well away from you while you sleep. Leave your phone on charge in the kitchen and take a step back in time by purchasing an analogue clock for your alarm.

Research has repeatedly shown that the blue light emission from screens will disturb your circadian rhythm (your body clock) and consequently your sleep. This is because blue light emission suppresses our melatonin levels, and melatonin's role is to signal us to sleep. So, when you find yourself using these devices at night, they are telling your brain it is daytime and not time to sleep. Think of blue light from screens working in the brain like a sunrise (which is also high in blue light) triggering you to wake up – not what you want before bed. Therefore, your bedroom is not a place for screens or work and must be completely dissociated from those sorts of activities; better still, you should replace full spectrum light bulbs with warm white bulbs or dimmers to further enhance the sleeping environment and minimise all blue light emission.

The second thing to consider is your bed quality. Your sleep is one of the most important aspects of your health, so don't be scared to spend some money on it. It is much more important to splash out on a good quality bed rather than a commodity you barely use and often pay more for. You spend approximately one-third of your day in bed – this is much more time than you probably spend commuting. So, when you can, invest in a good quality bed and pillow.

And the third thing you need to consider is your caffeine and alcohol intake. This means no caffeine (e.g. chocolate, cocoa, coffee, tea) within four to six hours of bed. For example, if you go to bed at 10pm, you should not have caffeine after 4pm. And despite most people thinking so, green tea and kombucha tea are not caffeine-free. The only tea that is caffeine-free is herbal tea, which is based on the herbal infusion from the leaves of the tree. Alcohol will also disrupt your sleep quality, so if you choose to drink, keep it to one self-pour drink per day (we tend to fill our glasses quite high, which equates closer to two standard drinks). You should also work towards a minimum of two alcohol-free days per week. Alcohol can still be part of your IWL plan (unless you are pregnant or breastfeeding) but you must realise that not only can it affect your sleep quality if you have too much, it can also make it more challenging to achieve weight loss on the weight-loss months if you are consuming more than one standard drink per night.

Our weakest time

As discussed in Chapter 9, the afternoons can be a very challenging time for most of us. The evenings are another challenging time – they are often when we find ourselves constantly craving an emotional high or wanting something to counter a low feeling of worthlessness after a stressful day. Typically, we associate this time with the couch and the TV as a method of unwinding, and we combat these feelings by reaching for food that makes us feel good – to give us that high. Known as comfort or emotional eating, this happens day after day, and is something that is quite challenging to gain control of. However, on the IWL plan, the evening is going to become one of the most productive times of the day, but there are two things you must do.

First, you must fix your food environment. If the block of chocolate is in the cupboard, you're more likely to eat it. It's less tempting when it's not in the home, and this will help guide you towards healthier choices. Remember, you should always *reach for nature first!* If your partner is the one to blame (that is, he or she is bringing chocolate into the house or eating it in front of you every evening), you need to discuss this, to get them aligned with your goals and new way of life. Better still, get your partner to read this book so s/he can provide support or so you can support one another every step of the way. Remember, if you're trying unsuccessfully to fall pregnant, a male partner is just as likely to be the reason for your fertility issues.

Second, you need to put together a to-do list of things that need addressing in the home or things you have long desired to try. Room by room, I want you to add each one to your to-do list, so that each evening you find yourself using free time constructively rather than destructively. This list shouldn't just be limited to chores around the house, it can also involve self-development tasks. For example, writing a letter to someone you haven't spoken to for a long time, painting a picture, volunteering in your community, or learning a new skill such as a language or playing a musical instrument. The evenings are some of the most challenging times for many of us, and by working through your to-do list at this time of the day or engaging in other activities such as a hobby (for example, building something with the kids or reading) you will stay occupied and less likely to reach for those comfort foods. This doesn't mean you can't still watch your favourite show on the couch, but it does mean you need to reduce the frequency of doing so. Just like the number of treats and takeaway foods you might be eating, you need to work towards reducing the frequency, and in this case, the number of TV viewing hours (three TV-free days per week and no more than two hours of TV on the other four days) to achieve a healthy balance. It's amazing what can be done at this time of the day if you put your mind to it, and if it's sleep deprivation you are managing, you must change your routine and go to bed earlier.

Where to start

Write your own to-do list, adding anything that you want to achieve. You will use this list at your weakest time, in the afternoon and evening. It might be an overdue task such as cleaning the windows or going through your wardrobe, drawer by drawer, or perhaps it's preparing the room for the baby you are planning to have or helping your kids build the cubby house or veggie garden you promised.

You can include on your to-do list all your rooms, cupboards and drawers that need clearing out, as well as the garage or storage rooms if you have them. Break each room down into as many jobs as possible, otherwise it can seem overwhelming. For example, it is much more manageable to go through a drawer rather than a whole cupboard at one time. This will allow you to clear out the house section by section and will give you a sense of reward when you tick something off.

And don't forget the bedroom and living room. You need to remove the TV and computer and any other technology from the bedroom. If you have a piece of cardio equipment (such as a stationary bike or a treadmill), put it in front of the TV.

Remember, this is a long game and not something that is achieved overnight. The more things on your list the better!

One of the key essentials to the IWL plan is leading a stream-lined yet well-organised life. On the IWL plan, as we have already discussed, there are foods that the body needs and there are those that need to be limited. The same goes for the materialistic posses-sions that we surround ourselves with. Holding on to all these things in life will not allow you to move on and break through into your new self. It is important to let go of your old life, your old notions of the size you should be, your notions of a fashion ideal that never suited your body shape in the first place and anything that is a reminder of the old you. This will allow you to break through the wall and into your inner silhouette – the weight your body wants to be. For example, all those clothes you have been holding on to all these years in the hope that you will one day fit into them when you lose weight. You will find it much harder to succeed if you continue to attach your success to weight loss, so going through all your clothes is one of the first things that needs to be on your to-do list. Every item that you haven't worn for six months must go into the clothing bin, to someone in need. And if it's not in good enough condition for charity (the last thing they need is junk), turn it into rags and use them for cleaning the house. The great thing is you can then re-use these rags repeatedly, simply by washing them in the machine after each use. When going through your clothes, there are no 'what ifs' and holding on to items in the hope you can re-wear them when you get to your new set point. Get rid of things wisely and reward yourself with a trip to the shops when you reach your new set point in the months to come.

The great thing about decluttering is that it keeps you engaged in constructive activities. While you are doing it, you are succeeding on the IWL plan because it will prevent you from sitting in front of the TV and engaging in activities you are not even aware of, like mindlessly devouring an entire block of chocolate. And if you really want to watch your favourite TV show you still can, but you must do it on the stationary bike that is now positioned in front of it or in the background as you undertake chores such as decluttering, packing the dishwasher or ironing. You will only break an old habit if you replace it with a new, positive one.

If you just don't feel like doing anything from time to time, this is fine too. In many instances, especially if you're a busy mum, the last thing you want to do at the end of the day is more work. After all, you've spent your entire day looking after the kids. In this instance, you still need to have a plan in place to prevent comfort eating. It might just mean treating yourself to a bubble bath with some soothing music and candles. A lot of the IWL community also use meditation. This is a training technique that anyone can do, to bring you back into the present moment and to guide your thoughts in a more constructive direction. Simply find a quiet place to sit – either on the floor cross-legged if you can or on a comfortable chair with your feet on the floor – and listen to your breathing. Take deep breaths in and out for a few minutes, building it up over time to 10 minutes a day. There are also plenty of wonderful meditation apps and you will find some great suggestions in the 'IWL Community' Facebook group.

Your task

Put together a to-do list and keep it in a place that is highly visible and handy so you can continually update it. Use the template on page 175 as a starting point. Whenever something pops into your head that needs to be actioned, write it on this list. This will be a big list and should be something you always keep visible. Some examples of things for your list could include cleaning out the fridge, dusting the blades on your ceiling fans, cleaning out your child's toy box, and so on.

Some tasks can be quite overwhelming, so make sure to break big tasks up into steps. For example, instead of writing 'Go through wardrobe', break it up into milestones such as 'Clean out the top drawer of the wardrobe', 'Clean out the second drawer of the wardrobe', and so on, until it appears manageable and achievable. There is no better feeling than being able to cross something off a list, so make sure each task is broken down into small jobs. The more you break down each task, the better.

To-do list

Examples

Clean kitchen drawers – top drawer ☐
Second drawer ☐
Third drawer ☐
Bottom drawer ☐
Clean out top drawer of wardrobe ☐
Clean out sock drawer ☐
Prepare ceiling bathroom for painting ☐
Paint ceiling bathroom first coat ☐
Paint ceiling bathroom second coat ☐

_____ ☐

_____ ☐

_____ ☐

_____ ☐

_____ ☐

_____ ☐

_____ ☐

_____ ☐

_____ ☐

CHAPTER 12

IMPLEMENTING THE IWL PLAN

I have now equipped you with the six principles of the IWL plan. They should be forefront in your mind and you should be able to recite them without even thinking about it. If you haven't already, go to the Interval Weight Loss website and explore the resources available to you. For a more guided approach, you can sign up to the Interval Weight Loss online program, but you can succeed exclusively with this book. The online program will also provide you access to the IWL community, where you can introduce yourself to other members of the IWL community and tell them about your long-term commitment to the plan. You will find other members in similar situations to you; it might be simply escaping from the yo-yo diet merry-go-round, losing weight so you can fall pregnant, trying to lose weight post-pregnancy, juggling a busy life with kids, struggling with menopause, or leading the life of a retiree – there will be someone you can connect with, someone who has been through your situation and can help you succeed.

The IWL plan never leaves you in the lurch – this is a way of life and if you apply the six principles you will always remember what you are trying to achieve.

In this chapter I will summarise what you need to be doing for the weight-loss and weight-maintenance months. The first few months are the most challenging as you come to terms with what routine works best for you and how to streamline your planning.

The weight-loss months will require you to eat at home more diligently and to include more physical activity in your daily routine, and the weight-maintenance months will allow you to relax a little with your food (and maybe even alcohol) intake while reducing the intensity of your exercise routine. You need to devote time to food shopping once per week so that you never run out of food, otherwise you will end up succumbing to the pressure of the vending machine, the impulse buy at the corner store or the Uber Eats takeaway meal. You need to plan each day and use to-do lists, but these will soon become second nature to you. Planning shouldn't feel arduous, but it needs your attention.

Regardless of whether you are in a weight-loss or weight-maintenance month, you must always follow the six principles of the IWL plan. As well as the six principles, the following tips will help keep you on track during the weight-loss months.

1. Eat five meals per day – the biggest meal when you get up and the smallest meal at the end of the day.

2. Wait at least 10 minutes after every meal and if you're still hungry you can then go back for more.

3. Eat home-cooked meals at least six days per week – use left-overs each night for lunch the next day to make it simple and save yourself time and money.

4. Allow yourself one treat food per week (for example, an ice-cream) and one takeaway or dining-out meal (for example, pizza).

5. Allow yourself one self-pour glass of alcohol per day, with at least two alcohol-free days per week. (The exception is if you are pregnant or breastfeeding. In this instance, you need to abstain from alcohol.) Alcohol consumption may require a lot of tweaking in the weight-loss months.

6. Drink a glass of water before every meal.

7. Do thirty minutes of structured exercise each day, of varying intensity and different types of activity.

8. Sleep for six to eight hours per night.

9. Have three TV-free days per week.

10. Watch no more than two hours of TV per day on the other four days.

You'll see that points nine and ten refer to TV viewing. For many, TV is an addiction and therefore this goal might be challenging at first. In practical terms, if you have a TV addiction, this means choosing your favourite shows and slowly reducing the amount of TV viewing by weaning yourself off gradually, to work towards the goal of three TV-free days per week. And recall that the only way to change a habit is to replace it with another. This will mean getting out your to-do list every night to keep yourself busy on something other than watching TV.

During the weight-maintenance months, the implementation of the IWL plan stays the same. There are some minor tweaks, specifically relating to the allowance of treats and takeaway meals, as well as the exercise prescription. The following is very similar to the one you have just seen, with a few minor changes.

1. Eat five meals per day – the biggest meal at the start and smallest meal at the end of the day (note that there is no difference in portion size to the weight-loss month).

2. Wait at least 10 minutes after every meal and if you're still hungry you can then go back for more.

3. Eat home-cooked meals at least five days per week – use leftovers each night for lunch the next day to make it simple and save yourself time and money.

4. Allow yourself two treat foods and two dining-out meals per week (if you can afford it). This can be substituted by cooking a treat meal at home.

5. Allow yourself one self-pour glass of alcohol per day. (The exception is if you are pregnant or breastfeeding. In this instance, you need to abstain from alcohol.) As with the weight-loss months, alcohol consumption may require some tweaking in the weight-maintenance months.

6. Drink a glass of water before every meal.

7. Do thirty minutes each day of structured exercise, of low to moderate intensity, without a need to vary the type of activity each day.

8. Sleep for six to eight hours per night.

9. Have two TV-free days per week.

10. Watch no more than two hours of TV per day on the other five days.

EXAMPLE WEEK OF A WEIGHT-LOSS MONTH

The most important thing to remember is that the following examples are just a guide, to give you an idea of how the IWL plan looks in practice and to show you how you might organise your week so you can give yourself the best possible chance on the plan. The first one is an example week from a weight-loss month of the IWL plan to suggest how you might structure your day. Recall that the IWL plan is a descriptive rather than prescriptive approach, and the beauty of the IWL plan is that it can be customised according to your personal needs. For example, a mum of two kids will have a very different schedule to a new grad lawyer or a retiree. You can, and should, make your own weekly IWL plan that fits your schedule, your priorities, your exercise preferences and your dietary requirements. But the underpinning principles of the IWL plan remain the same for everyone.

The first thing to add to your weekly calendar is your structured exercise routine. Guidelines for general health say you need to be doing at least five 30-minute exercise sessions per week (this can be brisk walking) and two days of body-strengthening exercises. You need to work out how that fits into your lifestyle and you need to mix up the duration, type and intensity of exercise to ensure you achieve your weight-loss goal during the weight-loss months.

The second thing to add to your calendar are social functions or catch-ups that you have for the week to account for your allowance of dining out/takeaway meals.

With the plan that follows, each day will also be accompanied by a large morning tea and small afternoon tea to ensure you have five meals per day. These meals can be selected from the selection of snacks and sides listed on pp. 345–349.

Lastly, this weekly plan includes reference to some of the recipes at the back of this book. You don't have to stick to these recipes; they're simply there to emphasise the type of ingredients you should use as the foundations for all recipes, and to show you how easy it is to cook. The recipes are designed specifically to be simple and are aimed at the time-poor who can't be in the supermarket and kitchen all night. If you want more ideas and inspiration, you will find recipes in the online program and the 'IWL Community' Facebook group, where members often share their own creations.

Sunday

In our household, we walk to the bakery first thing on a Sunday morning and grab a loaf of bread and the newspaper. After a leisurely morning at home and a large breakfast, we then go grocery shopping and get organised for the week (refer to the third principle of the IWL plan – *Full rainbow* – for a detailed grocery list that you can use as the basis of your shopping). Quite often we ride to the shops, because we have large baskets on the back of our bikes, but this is not always practical when doing a large shop for heavier items. It is something kids love as well. Our exercise on the weekends tends to be social. We try to do something new, whether that be going on a bushwalk we haven't tried before, doing laps in a different pool, or a different ocean swim or catching up with friends at the beach.

It's also a day when we tend to do a lot of housework, do some gardening and cook something that we can use for batches during the week. Even if we cook just a large batch of brown rice, it saves time in the kitchen each night. Or if you are cooking, say, two serves of quinoa or baking some roast veggies for a recipe, cook extra and freeze the rest for emergency meals or lunches through-out the week.

The following is a sample Sunday.

Brekkie: Eggs with sautéed spinach and avocado on two slices of wholegrain toast, and a skim-milk coffee. The perfect breakfast while reading the paper.

Morning tea: Refer to page 349 for a list of suitable snacks.

Lunch: Wholegrain sandwich with chicken, avocado and salad.

Afternoon tea: Refer to page 349 for a list of suitable snacks.

Dinner: Andrew's chicken enchiladas (page 309).

Hot tip: make double the serving and enjoy for lunch on Monday instead of spending your Sunday meal-prepping.

After dinner: Work through your to-do list, because this helps to keep your mind occupied and not thinking about food. To-do lists keep you organised and constructive.

Bed: Go to bed early and read. Preferably 10pm for eight hours' sleep. You could also try listening to relaxation music, practising meditation or listening to a podcast, especially if you have trouble drifting off to sleep. Be mindful of what devices you are using to ensure you are adhering to the sixth principle of the IWL plan – *No blue light after twilight.*

Monday

Start your week off the right way by getting up 30 minutes earlier than normal. Instead of getting off the bus or train at your usual stop, get off earlier and walk. These small changes to your day will help you get to the minimum 10,000 steps per day. One kilometre of walking is approximately 1300 steps, and of course this varies depending on your height and stride length, but it gives you an idea of how many kilometres you need to do to get to 10,000 steps per day (approximately 8 kilometres). And it doesn't have to be walking; it can be bike riding or swimming, which is strongly recommended when first starting out on your IWL plan.

Brekkie: Muesli with yoghurt, berries, honey and milk.

Morning tea: Refer to page 349 for a list of suitable snacks.

Lunch: Leftovers from the night before.

Afternoon tea: Refer to page 349 for a list of suitable snacks.

Dinner: San choy bau (page 317).

After dinner: An evening stroll around the block or a 30-minute cycle on the bike while watching a favourite TV show.

Bed: Get into bed by 10pm and read. You are aiming for eight hours' rest each night on the IWL plan.

Tuesday

Brekkie: Avocado on two slices of wholegrain toast with skim-milk coffee + 200 gram tub of yoghurt.

Morning tea: Refer to page 349 for a list of suitable snacks.

Lunch: Lunch prepared from Sunday that was in the freezer or leftovers from Monday's dinner.

Go for a lunchtime walk or run. On time-poor days make it a HIIT session and on other days make it a continuous aerobic session. It really doesn't matter what you do when it comes to exercise. I just want you to be moving and engaging in something you enjoy. And it needs to be gradual. If you come out of the gates blazing, you will get injured or burn yourself out. Remember, this is *not* an all-or-nothing approach.

Afternoon tea: Refer to page 349 for a list of suitable snacks.

Dinner: Calamari with potato salad (page 326).

After dinner: Get out a board game, help the kids with their homework or work on your to-do list. Everyone's lifestyle is different. The main thing is to keep busy because if the evening time is used constructively you will avoid reaching for that block of chocolate.

Bed: Get into bed by 10pm and read.

Wednesday

Brekkie: Oats with fruit, honey and yoghurt.

Morning tea: Refer to page 349 for a list of suitable snacks.

Lunch: Leftovers from the night before.

Afternoon tea: Refer to page 349 for a list of suitable snacks.

Dinner: Ginger and miso marinated chicken with charred broccolini (page 321).

After dinner: During daylight savings we use the evening time to get outdoors to do some gardening, or other work around the house. If you have kids, get them involved.

Bed: 10pm for eight hours' sleep.

Who says you need to save your dining out or takeaway meal for the weekend? Wednesday is often a great night of the week to go out with friends or family because it's less crowded and there are usually plenty of mid-week specials. Having it mid-week is also a wonderful idea because you often have more time on Friday, Saturday or Sunday night to prepare a great home-cooked meal. This is the one time of the week you can break the chopstick rule unless, of course, you are eating Asian cuisine. Order a few plates to share, which will help reduce your portion size. If there are leftovers, you can take them home for lunch the next day.

Thursday

Brekkie: Go for a morning walk or jump on the exercise bike for 30 minutes. It's a great way to get in a quick 4000 steps before work. Have a simple breakfast such as wholegrain toast with avocado and tomato (we keep our bread in the freezer and get it out as we need it) with a 200-gram tub of yoghurt and fruit.

Morning tea: Refer to page 349 for a list of suitable snacks.

Lunch: Leftovers from the evening before or a meal from the freezer if you went out.

Afternoon tea: Refer to page 349 for a list of suitable snacks.

Have you tried walking meetings? Who says meetings need to be in an office sitting down? Whenever possible, it's something I like to implement to get up my steps throughout the day. Getting outside is also more conducive to creativity.

Dinner: Fish tacos (page 318).

After dinner: If you've been on your feet all day and have hit your exercise goal, relax. Try using a journal to record your thoughts and progress on the IWL plan. It's a wonderful way to reflect on your wins and barriers yet to overcome.

Bed: 10pm for eight hours' sleep. Remember, your sleep quality is not going to change overnight and it will require persistence until everything falls into place.

Friday

Brekkie: Overnight oats with fruit and yoghurt, plus wholegrain toast with peanut butter.

Don't forget to keep mixing up your exercise variety and to include a day of non-body weight bearing exercise every second day.

Maybe it's practical to try riding your bike to work or leaving the car at home on some days and walking? Whatever it may be, it's likely you need to think of ways to change your daily routine so that you are getting in more incidental activity.

Morning tea: Refer to page 349 for a list of suitable snacks.

Lunch: Leftovers from the night before.

Afternoon tea: Refer to page 349 for a list of suitable snacks.

Dinner: If you didn't eat out on Wednesday, you might want to go out tonight. Make sure your dining out or takeaway meal is something you love. I don't want you to be perusing the menu for healthier options. If you love the laksa, get the laksa.

Treat: Much like your takeaway meal, have whatever you like. I love gelato!

Saturday

Brekkie: We typically do a big breakfast cook-up on a Saturday utilising plenty of vegetables from the garden. Breakfast is a great way to get in veggies, and if you don't it can be challenging to meet the recommended five serves of veg every day. Pan-fry some eggs with broccolini, mushrooms and spinach with a little garlic and soy sauce and have with a couple of slices of wholegrain toast.

Morning tea: Refer to page 349 for a list of suitable snacks.

Lunch: Toasted sandwich.

Afternoon tea: Refer to page 349 for a list of suitable snacks.

Dinner: Because we have more time on our hands on the weekend, we typically use this time to trial a new recipe. We also like to have barbecues and go for picnics whenever we can.

EXAMPLE WEEK OF A WEIGHT-MAINTENANCE MONTH

This is a sample week from a weight-maintenance month of IWL. As per the weekly plan provided for the weight-loss month, it's just a guide and needs to be adapted to your lifestyle.

As per the weight-loss months, the first thing you need to add to your calendar is your structured exercise routine. If it's in the calendar, there is no excuse that you don't have time to do it. Your health is far more important than filling your calendar with meetings that you probably didn't need anyway. During the weight-maintenance months you can allow yourself a little more flexibility; you don't need to worry about varying it up, you simply need to keep up the exercise.

The second thing to add to your calendar is any social functions or catch-ups that you have for the week to account for your allowance of dining out/takeaway meals.

Your portion sizes stay the same during the weight-maintenance months, but you can enjoy more dining out, takeaway meals and treats. Most people in the IWL community also report a slightly greater allowance for alcohol during the weight-maintenance months. This will require some trial and error to see how your weight tracks from week to week. The first few months are always the most challenging on the IWL plan as you learn to master your body's responses to the small changes you make.

You are required to stick to five meals a day. And as per the weight-loss months, your morning and afternoon tea meals can be selected from page 349.

Sunday

Brekkie: Sunday is a great day to devote a little more time to breakfast. We love going for a morning walk first thing to grab the newspaper and a loaf of bread from our local baker. And then we usually cook up a variety of veggies with some eggs to go on our freshly baked wholegrain bread.

Morning tea: Refer to page 349 for a list of suitable snacks.

Lunch: Japanese prawn pancakes (page 293).

Go for a long walk or attend a class at your gym. This is a day of the week when you typically have more time on your hands, so make the most of it and get moving.

Afternoon tea: Refer to page 349 for a list of suitable snacks.

Dinner: Broccolini and edamame salad with sesame dressing (page 292).

After dinner: Relax and watch that TV series you've been dying to catch up on, or read.

Bed: 10pm for eight hours' sleep. The same sleep routine must apply during the weight-maintenance months; you must establish what works for you to help you wind down and drift off to sleep.

Monday

The weight-maintenance months are not about sweat and variety of exercise. Your weight won't go up if you keep moving. Make sure to keep up the incidental activity by walking to a bus or train stop that you typically wouldn't. If you drive, try parking further away or going for a stroll before you sit down at your desk. Every little bit of movement adds up.

Brekkie: Overnight oats (page 281).

Morning tea: Refer to page 349 for a list of suitable snacks.

Lunch: Leftovers from the night before.

Afternoon tea: Refer to page 349 for a list of suitable snacks.

Dinner: Miso fried rice (page 307).

After dinner: Get out your to-do list and keep busy. Remember, this is often the weakest time of the day and you need to break your old routine and form a new one.

Bed: 10pm for eight hours' sleep. If your sleep isn't improving, try something different such as reorienting your room, because often physical change can be enough to break through a mental barrier.

Tuesday

Brekkie: Homemade muesli: oats, dry roasted nuts, berries, cinnamon, honey and milk.

Set your alarm 15 minutes earlier than usual and go for a quick walk or pedal on your bike.

Morning tea: Refer to page 349 for a list of suitable snacks.

Lunch: Leftovers from the evening before or a meal from the freezer.

For many people who lead a very busy work life, it is vital to make use of lunchtime for structured activity. Schedule some time in your calendar to allow for a good hit out (a walk, run, swim or gym workout) and some lunch.

Afternoon tea: Refer to page 349 for a list of suitable snacks.

Dinner: Go to the movies and enjoy one of your two dining-out allowances for the week. Or stay at home, order some takeaway and put on a movie. Be mindful of how much you order and try to put some aside for leftovers the next day. When you're at home, you can always use your chopsticks.

Bed: 10pm for eight hours' sleep.

Wednesday

Brekkie: Oats with berries and milk with a side of yoghurt and fruit.

Morning tea: Refer to page 349 for a list of suitable snacks.

Lunch: Leftovers from the batch-cooking meal you prepared on Sunday and placed in the freezer.

Afternoon tea: Refer to page 349 for a list of suitable snacks.

Dinner: Pesto chicken with pasta (page 336).

After dinner: Work on your hobby, get out your to-do list, or help the kids with some of their homework.

Bed: 10pm for eight hours' sleep.

Thursday

Brekkie: Wholegrain toast with avocado and tomato, a piece of fruit and a 200 g tub of yoghurt.

Morning tea: Refer to page 349 for a list of suitable snacks.

Lunch: Leftovers from the night before.

Afternoon tea: Refer to page 349 for a list of suitable snacks.

Dinner: Green spring-y salad (page 289).

After dinner: Is there a stationary bike in your garage collecting dust? Get it out and stick it in front of the TV. Exercising in front of the TV is a good way to get moving and prevent yourself comfort eating in front of the screen.

Bed: Midnight for six hours' sleep. If you have a social function to attend, it's not always practical to get to bed early enough for eight hours of sleep. Remember, the goal is for six to eight hours per night and it is about the quality not the quantity.

Friday

Brekkie: Homemade muesli: oats, nuts, berries, cinnamon, honey and milk.

Keep an eye on your incidental activity for the week by checking over the data on your exercise-tracking device. If you're not meeting your targets, you need to think about where you can get in more exercise throughout your day. For example, using the stairs instead of the lift and banning use of the car whenever possible.

Morning tea: Refer to page 349 for a list of suitable snacks.

Lunch: Leftovers from the night before.

Afternoon tea: Refer to page 349 for a list of suitable snacks.

Dinner: Roasted eggplant with pine nut salsa (page 303).

Saturday

Brekkie: Wholegrain toast with fried egg, avocado and tomato.

Morning tea: Refer to page 349 for a list of suitable snacks.

Lunch: Cauliflower and pomegranate salad (page 291) or if on the go, make a toasted sandwich.

Afternoon tea: Refer to page 349 for a list of suitable snacks.

Evening: Go out with friends and enjoy your second dining-out meal of the week. One of the most loved things about the IWL plan is that it is real. You don't have to avoid a social function or worry about what restaurant your friends have picked because of the risk of jeopardising your diet. You can have anything on the IWL plan, so go out and enjoy yourself. The thing you do need to do is plan as best you can for your allowance of dining-out and takeaway meals per week. This will be an ongoing task to ensure you don't overcommit yourself with social gatherings centred around food eaten away from home.

CHAPTER 13

YOU CAN CHANGE YOUR BODY

Years of stress on the body caused by dieting will result in your body becoming very resistant to change. Those who are first timers at weight loss will always respond more quickly than someone who has previously dieted. Refer to the start of the book where I taught you about the biological protections that kick into gear with weight loss. Well, with every diet you follow, your body becomes better at resisting change, hence you find it harder and harder to lose weight with each subsequent dieting attempt.

But the good news is you *can* overcome this resistance to change. I know that many of you might be worried about your biological clock and feel a sense of urgency to lose weight right away. And, yes, it may take you a little longer to start losing weight than someone that has never dieted, but a couple of minor tweaks will get the results you're after. The one thing I ask of you is to be patient. A couple of months is not going to make a big difference on your ability to conceive. I *will* get you losing weight.

Your diet type

Having a better understanding of your personal triggers and daily habits will help increase your chance of success on the IWL plan and set you up for long-term success. Knowing your personal diet type – there are five of them – is one way of better understanding these personal triggers and help you lose the required 2 kilograms in the weight-loss months. Most people fall into either 'the thinker' or 'the craver' diet types.

The Thinker – The thinker constantly overthinks and worries about failure, which leads to stress and a derailing of progress. They tend to give up when things get challenging. If you fall into this category, it is important to not be hard on yourself. We all have slip-ups with our food. And most importantly, don't get caught up in the small stuff – in this book I'm giving you all the information to succeed on your weight-loss journey, but you do need to read it over and over again to engrain the six principles of the IWL plan and unlearn all the wrong information you have been told.

The Craver – The craver is always on the search for delicious food. They find it hard to stop when they get their hands on it, which leads to overeating. If this is you, you must ensure that hunger never sets in, to prevent that all-too-common scenario where you skip meals, find yourself ravenous and then end up reaching for anything you can get your hands on. Going to the supermarket after eating (preferably breakfast, which is the biggest meal of the day) is also wise to prevent yourself loading the trolley with chocolate, chips and sweets.

The Socialiser – The socialiser needs a plan that is flexible because they won't let food restrictions stifle their social life. As you will know by now, nothing is off limits with the IWL plan. You can include all foods and your favourite meals in this plan. If you are a keen socialiser, make the shift to social events that are not based around food and alcohol. For example, go for a walk instead of sitting at the cafe with banana bread. When you're going out, try to pick a healthier option at the venue, or a healthier cuisine – think Hawaiian poke bowls or Greek rather than dumplings or pizza.

The Foodie – The foodie has a fondness for making, eating and experiencing food. Much like the socialiser, it's great news for you as well. A lot of baby boomers tend to fall into 'the socialiser' or 'the foodie' diet type, and the IWL plan ticks all your boxes. This plan doesn't require you to eat specially formulated foods or shakes. It brings the pleasure back to food. It encourages you to cook, but it may require a slight change in your cooking preferences and the ingredients you use. You can still entertain all your guests as frequently as you like, and you can do it with your favourite IWL recipes. Don't feel like you're restricted to the recipes in this book and its predecessors – there are literally thousands of recipes out there that are appropriate to the IWL lifestyle.

The Freewheeler – The freewheeler tends to make spontaneous and impulsive food choices and finds planning the hardest aspect when it comes to meals. If you fall into this diet type personality, you are probably still asking, 'Where is my meal plan?' or 'How many calories do I need to eat?' and might struggle at first with the concept of not being provided with this structure and a strict set of rules. Yes, you still need to plan to succeed on the IWL plan, but it doesn't require you to wander the supermarket for hours looking for obscure ingredients or see you in the kitchen all night cooking. With the IWL plan, cooking is fun, quick and easy. You just need to grocery shop once per week, and your favourite recipes can be on regular rotation. The biggest part of your planning is remembering to eat frequently, so you must take food with you to avoid impulse buys.

If you are not seeing any change on the scales during the weight-loss months, this could be for many reasons. These are the common ones to look out for (not in any given order, because everyone is different).

- ☐ Lack of exercise variety – it must be completely different to your weight-maintenance months.
- ☐ Not hitting 10,000 steps per day.
- ☐ Not using a device to monitor your activity level – neglecting to write down your steps or electronically tracking your activity every day.
- ☐ Too many 'treat' foods – more than one per week.
- ☐ Dining out or getting takeaway too often – more than once per week.
- ☐ Not eating five meals per day – skipping meals regularly only to overeat at the next meal time.
- ☐ Not eating enough – not seeing the weight change on the scales and restricting food intake as a result.
- ☐ Not having enough plant-based meals (not everything needs to be meat).
- ☐ Having more than one self-pour glass of alcohol per day and/or fewer than two alcohol-free days per week.

☐ Not making sure most of your food intake is at the start of the day – failing to make breakfast the biggest meal of the day only to overeat in the afternoon and evening.

☐ Eating too fast – failing to eat with chopsticks.

☐ Eating when not hungry – failing to have a glass of water before every meal or before each sensation of hunger, particularly after dinner.

☐ Not eating at the dinner table and away from technological distraction.

☐ Not using a bread-and-butter plate or rice bowl for the evening meal.

☐ Not making the time to prepare evening meals – eating homemade meals fewer than six days per week.

☐ Watching TV and mindlessly snacking, scrolling through social media – more than one hour per day.

☐ Lack of sleep and failing to turn the blue light off after twilight – getting fewer than six hours' sleep per night.

☐ Going to bed too late – staying up after 10pm in front of the TV.

☐ Failing to plan your day – overlooking the importance of scheduling every day (the night before or the morning of).

☐ Failing to use a to-do list – not writing things down as they pop into your head.

Use this checklist as a prompt every time you commence a weight-loss month. If you are convinced that you are successfully putting all these strategies into practice and you still don't see the weight budging on the scales, don't panic. The worst thing you can do is reduce food intake thinking that is the cause of your problems. Often it is the opposite, and you may need to focus on increasing the amount of wholesome and nutritious food you eat (see the list of foods outlined in the third principle of the IWL plan – *Full rainbow*). Depriving your body of good nutrition will only result in your body shutting down. You just need to make sure you are keeping the less nutritious and white, refined sources of carbohydrate to a minimum (including all those foods we think are healthy, such as muffins and banana bread) of once per week.

Many of those who struggle to lose weight have benefitted greatly from the use of a food journal. It's a good way to monitor how many of those treat foods you are eating, while also monitoring how your appetite changes throughout the day. I suggest keeping a food diary for a month, paying specific attention to the following.

1. Keeping the 'treats' to a maximum of once per week.

2. Keeping takeaway and dining out to once per week.

3. Ensuring that you are having five meals per day.

4. Substituting many of your meat-based meals with legumes, tofu or eggs as the protein source.

5. Remembering to focus most of your food intake at the start of the day.

Here are the steps to follow when recording in a food journal.

1. Highlight when 'treat' foods appear in your journal. If it is currently five per week, reduce to four treats, until you work your way to one per week on the weight-loss months. Don't eliminate the treat foods altogether – it takes time to retrain your brain and 66 days to break a habit.

2. Highlight when takeaway or dining-out meals appear in your journal. Reduce gradually until you achieve one takeaway or dining-out meal per week on the weight-loss months. Don't eliminate eating out altogether, unless you

can't afford it – it is something that should be enjoyed and still be part of a healthy lifestyle.

3. Count the number of meals per day from breakfast through to dinner to ensure you are having enough. Dessert is not included in this count (you don't need it if you follow the IWL plan properly). The only exception is if you want to include dessert as one of your treats per week. You must have five meals per day (refer to my sample weekly plans).

4. Pay attention to afternoon and evening snacking. You might find that you are still subconsciously eating after dinner even though you're not even hungry. Worse still, it may not be the healthy foods you are advised to snack on (refer to the third principle of the IWL plan – *Full rainbow*).

5. Highlight the number of meat-based meals you are consuming. Not every meal needs to contain meat and by including more vegetarian and plant-based options, you will improve your gut microbiome through the increased fibre intake and also heighten your chance of kickstarting a weight-loss phase. While on this topic, don't get caught up in all those cleverly marketed 'gut-friendly' diets you see on the shelves – they're nothing more than an eating plan that tells you to have more of the very foods that are prescribed in the IWL plan – plenty of foods rich is fibre (soluble fibre, insoluble fibre and resistant starch).

6. Record your hunger scale before and after meals to ensure you are seeing a decrease in hunger before meals towards the end of the day. This will only happen if you have most of your food intake at the start of the day. Use the following hunger scale previously discussed to monitor your appetite.

-1	0	1	2	3	4
Full and uncomfortable	Not at all hungry	Satisfied	Slightly hungry	Somewhat hungry	Hungry

The common mistake

Many people who start the IWL plan believe they are already active and fail to measure their daily movement. I would strongly recommend investing in an activity monitor to see how much activity you are currently doing. If you are meeting your goals, then great, but if you're not, the first thing to work on is increasing your incidental activity. But as previously explained, you must be very mindful of preventing setback through injury. For those who are meeting their goals and still not losing weight, this doesn't mean you have to increase your activity level, but it does mean you need to vary the type of exercise you are doing to ensure you incorporate a range of different exercise intensities throughout the week.

For example, if you currently go to the gym three days a week, the pool one day, and you walk around the neighbourhood on the other three days, there are a few changes you could make. You could change the days you are doing each type of activity, you could change the type of exercise you are doing and you could change the intensities of the activities you are doing. For example, you could try doing some new classes at the gym, you could do some HIIT training in the pool, or you could explore a different walking route.

Lastly, if you are convinced that your food intake and activity routine is in accordance with all six principles of the IWL plan, focus on improving your sleep, by trying different strategies to help you drift off. Anything that doesn't involve your phone. Sleep plays a vital role in weight management and the more you can get, the better off you will be. It may just mean more rest rather than sleep per se, so make sure to keep a routine in place whereby you go to bed at the same time and wake at the same time each day.

If you don't lose weight in any given weight-loss month, don't worry, just move on to the weight-maintenance month. Don't keep trying to play catch up and don't continue trying to lose weight. Give your body a break and hit it with a new stress (for example, change in exercise intensity) after the weight-maintenance month is over.

CHAPTER 14

THE IMPORTANCE OF DIET BREAKS

It's a wonderful feeling to see the weight coming off on the scales, but you still need to ensure you follow the first principle of the IWL plan – *You can't fight evolution* – by putting on the brakes every second month. This will allow your body to recalibrate at its new set point along the way. I can't stress this enough. The race to fall pregnant or wind back the clock often means people get excited when they see the number decreasing on the scales and consequently continue to lose weight. This won't help you fall pregnant quicker and it's only going to see you regain weight in the long term due to strong biological forces that will come into play.

If you're frustrated by the notion of having to impose diet breaks or are losing the weight too quickly, I'm sorry to say you will fail, because you are disregarding the science behind the IWL plan. As blunt as it might sound, never think that success will result on this plan if you continue with weight loss during a weight-maintenance month. Your body will only fight the weight loss and you will fail long term – you will get the same result you always got: weight loss followed by weight regain. Every second month your body needs to rest and re-calibrate at its new set point (approximately 2 kilograms lighter each time).

One of the most rewarding aspects of translating a message on a large scale is when I hear from the people themselves. But the ones that stick with me the most are from those that I can tell haven't grasped a full understanding of the IWL plan, particularly relating to the first principle of the IWL plan – *You can't fight evolution*. This was particularly evident after the release of my first book and hence was something that needed to be better articulated in subsequent books, but in the meantime, I had to ensure these people understood the plan, so they didn't end up with the same old result they had always got. One of these community IWL members, whom I'll call Sarah, wrote:

'Hi Nick, I heard your interview on ABC radio and decided to buy your book. The plan has been going very well. I've lost about 8 kilograms in the last three months sticking to your plan and cutting out some foods that I know are not good. I have also started walking to work each day and believe it or not, it isn't much slower than catching the bus! The combination of a large breakfast, having a medium-sized lunch and a small dinner on a saucer is gold. Thank you.'

Immediately I was concerned by the amount of weight Sarah had lost to date, because the IWL plan allows a person to lose 8 kilograms over eight months, not three! This was only going to result in long-term pain and disappointment. The other red flag was the all-or-nothing approach to food. One of the most fulfilling principles of the IWL plan is that it allows you to eat whatever you want and certainly doesn't advocate completely cutting out certain foods. Science has proven that this doesn't work. We can all cut foods we love for a certain period (refer to Chapter 1 – our biological protections) but this all-or-nothing approach to weight

loss doesn't work because these foods give us pleasure. You
end up giving in to your cravings, which triggers a psychological response dubbed the 'what-the-hell effect' – a vicious
cycle of indulgence, followed by guilt, followed by greater
indulgence. You end up eating the whole cake instead of
just a slice. After I asked for some more details on Sarah's
approach and progress to date, she replied:

'I am aware I have probably lost a bit too much, it is hard
to stop when you see great results and I find it easier if I just
remove the foods that I love from my diet . . . I understand
your advice and will try to maintain for a month. Only
losing 2 kilograms every couple of months is not appealing
at all. I desperately want to fall pregnant.'

This clarified what I thought had taken place. Sarah had
not implemented the IWL plan as per the six principles.
Unfortunately, this was going to result in disappointment
at a later stage. First, the periods of weight maintenance had
not been implemented after each block of weight loss and
as a result, Sarah's body would already be starting to work
differently, to eliminate the stress and fight the 8 kilogram
weight loss. It was also going to see her going back for
her favourite foods after a period of complete avoidance. I
followed up a few months down the track, and Sarah sadly
reported:

'My progress has been average; I have regained most of
the weight I lost. I think the fact that I couldn't keep losing
weight messed with my head. I'm back onto the plan and
really want to get down to my goal weight.'

For Sarah, she hadn't yet escaped her dieting approach to
weight loss. After digging deeper into her background, I saw
that she had become obsessed with her body image and the
number on the scales, and the constant thought of dieting

had completely saturated her mindset for the past 10 years. Whenever she went out, she dined in fear that she would eat something that would be forbidden and would make her fat. Unfortunately, she saw the IWL plan as another diet and the 'quick fix' she was after. After I followed up with her again three months later, Sarah replied:

'Hi Nick, I've totally fallen off and back to where I started. I'm now reading your book again.'

The refreshing thing was that Sarah hadn't turned to the latest and greatest diet – she was now aware that those 28-day plans, 8-week or 12-week programs were not the answer and had only seen her worse off for going on them over the years. She had opened my book again and was re-reading it. I was ecstatic to hear this.

I'm not going to sugarcoat this. You too will end up like Sarah, unless you closely follow the six principles of the IWL plan:

You can't fight evolution
Reach for nature first
Full rainbow
Use chopsticks
Choose to move
No blue light after twilight

Only then will you achieve your goal weight loss without your body fighting itself.

Weight trajectory

Weight-loss trajectories are never perfect and some months you might lose a little more (for example 2.5 kilograms) and other months a little less (for example 1.5 kilograms). This is, of course, fine, but the goal must be to stick as close as possible to the 2 kilogram weight-loss prescription. The same can be said for the weight-maintenance months. If your weight is up by 0.3 kilograms or down by 0.4 kilograms over the course of the month, this is also fine. Again, stick as close as possible to maintaining the weight loss from the previous month.

As a rule of thumb, at the end of your weight-maintenance month the goal is to have kept within 1 kilogram of the previous month's weight. You will find it more realistic to keep within 0.5 kilograms if your starting weight is less than 100 kilograms, and more appropriate to keep within 1 kilogram if you starting weight is more than 100 kilograms. If your weight is down by 1 kilogram at the end of the weight-maintenance month, factor this in to your next month's weight loss, which would mean allowing another 1 kilogram (and not 2 kilograms) weight loss in the month that approaches. On the contrary, if your weight is up by 1 kilogram, factor this in to next month's weight-loss goal – aim to be 3 kilograms down at the end of the weight-loss month. It is a realistic goal to keep within 1 kilogram of your goal trajectory each month due to the huge variance that you see in body weight; all you are monitoring is the trend over time. Don't panic or put pressure on yourself if you don't see weight loss in a given month or the weight loss is less than the 2-kilogram goal. You will still get to your new goal set point.

Putting on the brakes

For some people, despite easing off and allowing more flexibility during the weight-maintenance month, their weight continues to go down. This is typical in those who have never or rarely dieted before and in those with larger starting body weights (greater than

100 kilograms) because they have a larger body mass to lose. If you have never dieted, your body will always respond faster to weight loss the first time around. It hasn't had the same stresses imposed on it compared to someone who has repeatedly dieted. If you find that your weight is still going down, there are a few things to look for to ensure you correct it. These are the common pitfalls:

1. Not allowing yourself 'treat' foods.

2. Not allowing yourself to eat out or have takeaway food.

3. Telling yourself that certain foods or drinks are forbidden.

4. Cutting carbs.

5. Being overly restrictive with food intake.

6. Counting calories.

7. Exercising too much.

8. Varying the type of exercise.

9. Not reducing the intensity of the exercise.

10. Not focusing on the long-term goal.

The good news is that it is an easy problem to fix and allows you to really take the accelerator off and relax. I stress, though, that it is a big problem and must be fixed – you must stop further weight loss from occurring. More than likely you are being overly restrictive with your food intake or not allowing yourself to enjoy your favourite 'treat' foods enough. Don't be restrictive in your food intake; keep the same food plan in place as the weight-loss and weight-maintenance months but allow an extra treat or two – a total of three treats per week on the weight-maintenance month instead of two. You also can allow an extra dining out or takeaway meal, bringing you to a total of three per week on the weight-maintenance months instead of two. If you really don't want to increase the number of treats or takeaway meals you eat – it might be for financial reasons or perhaps you've already made the successful transition to getting the same pleasure from nature's treats – I have some other healthy tips below. Following the IWL plan will be easy if you don't adopt the all-or-nothing approach that has always failed you in the past. If you stick to the plan and maintain your weight every second month you *will* succeed.

Incorporating healthy fats

If, for the reasons mentioned above, you are keeping your treats and takeaway meals to once per week, there are some other changes to your food plan that can be made. Specifically, you will need to include more 'good' fats in your daily eating plan. This means cooking with more extra-virgin olive oil than usual, putting more avocado on your toast, your sandwich or in your salad, or having two to three times the number of nuts and seeds that you usually have. These sources of fat are good for your heart health and the best way to increase your calorie intake to ensure you don't keep dropping weight on the scales.

Your exercise plan

The other thing to be conscious of is your exercise routine. This month is not about sweating it out. Remember, this is the month when you can relax a little and do the same thing. You shouldn't add new exercises or different types of exercise during a weight-maintenance month. This will also allow your body the rest it needs and ensure you reduce the possibility of injury. Just keep the same routine you had in place for the previous weight-loss month but with a focus on reduced intensity to only include low- to moderate-exertion activities.

Many people are also guilty of doing too much exercise. The weight-maintenance month is not a time to increase your activity volume, especially if you successfully lost weight the month prior. Even if you didn't lose weight in the prior month, the weight-maintenance months are not the time to be experimenting with your exercise. It's a time to relax and rest a little before ramping it up again in the next weight-loss month.

CHAPTER 15

WHAT TO DO WHEN YOU'VE REACHED YOUR GOAL WEIGHT

Getting to your realistic goal 'set point' is a huge achievement. Providing you have lost it in exactly the way prescribed in the IWL plan, you won't find your body starting to fight the weight loss. Unlike the end of a 28-day program, or an eight- or 12-week program, the IWL plan doesn't leave you in the lurch once you've reached your goal. You never stop following the IWL plan, because it becomes a way of life, but you can now take the focus off any further weight loss. If you happened to fall pregnant along the way, you must *not* continue to lose weight. You can recommence the weight-loss months after the delivery of your child.

When you reach your new set point, the focus stays on the weight-maintenance months. You continue to put everything into place that you have learnt – the new eating habits, regular exercise, productive use of time and better quality sleep. You keep following all six principles of the IWL plan and you keep monitoring your weight each week to ensure it stays the same. If you continue doing this, you will keep the weight off for life.

What if you want to set a new goal weight?

Let's imagine you have achieved the realistic goal weight loss that I helped you calculate at the start of the book. You feel great but still want to lose more. For many, it's not realistic or necessary to keep losing weight. But, for a few, it may be appropriate to do so. Whatever your situation may be, always remember that just a small amount of sustained weight loss (3 kilograms) results in all sorts of improvements in health parameters, as well as a significant reduction in the risk of dying from cardiovascular disease.

Recall Melissa and her husband from earlier in the book. Melissa's goal set point was 76 kilograms, a 16 kilogram weight loss. After a challenging start, mainly because she was fixated on what size portions and quantities she should be eating (a hangover from a long history of dieting), she started to get the hang of the IWL plan. Most importantly, she started to gain an appreciation for her appetite-hormone signalling and that weight trajectory is never as one hopes (that is, it rarely looks as pretty as a 2-kilogram drop in the weight-loss month, followed by a perfect month of weight maintenance, and so on). In fact, for the first three months she didn't lose anything, even though she was desperate to start losing weight in the hope it would help her fall pregnant again. Frustratingly for her, during the first two months of implementing the IWL plan she was still regaining weight as her body readjusted after coming off the keto diet. She came to understand there wasn't much she could do about this but by following the principles of the IWL plan she was giving her body the best chance at success. Luckily she managed to abstain from going on another diet during this frustrating time. Her weight plateaued towards the end of the second month, and during the third month, despite not losing any weight, she started to get joy out of how much better she was feeling and the fact that she was no longer having to cut out certain foods or food groups from her eating plan. After what ended up being a three-month wash-out period, her body then responded, and the weight started to drop. She lost the goal 16 kilograms over approximately three years (she had her second child during that time). She maintained this weight for another six months, before then going on to lose more weight. Melissa now weighs 70 kilograms (a total weight loss of 22 kilograms) and she has accepted that she needn't be back at 60 kilograms, where she was in her younger years. Her husband Pete also did very well, losing 10 kilograms over the year and then a further 4 kilograms over the second year. He now weighs 82 kilograms, which is very close to his lowest weight as an adult. Melissa and Pete are a great testament to how you can succeed on the IWL plan, especially when you are supported by a loved one. Despite Melissa thinking that she was the reason they couldn't conceive, it's just as likely that Pete was to blame – or the issue may be unconnected to weight. Obesity is one of the leading causes of infertility, however, and it's not always clear which partner's fertility is the issue. So, if your partner or husband is carrying a little extra weight, get him on the IWL plan as well. You will both benefit from not only the support you offer one another, but also the increased chance of being able to conceive a child.

Sneaky weight gain

One of the six principles of the IWL plan requires you to weigh yourself weekly. Even after reaching your goal weight, this is a habit that must continue for life. The pressures of work life, having more kids or getting older can make it very challenging to keep on top of your weight. You must keep tracking your weight and monitoring the trend over time. That way, if you notice your weight creeping up – more than 1 kilogram per year – you can make the necessary adjustments to get back on track. Perhaps you need to reinstate some of the key principles of the weight-loss months such as exercise variety and intensity and type of exercise. Or perhaps you notice a change in your food intake; for example, you've found yourself on the couch mindlessly eating more often, the frequency of treat foods or takeaway meals may have increased to more than once per week, you've been skipping breakfast or not having it as your biggest meal of the day, or the size of your evening meal has started to increase. Keeping a food journal will help you assess this as well as monitoring your hunger scale before and after meals.

What are the key aspects of successfully keeping the weight off long term?

1. Continuing to track your body weight each week and monitoring the trend over time. If your weight goes up by more than 1 kilogram over the year, you need to reinstate the aspects of the IWL plan weight-loss months.

2. Keeping a food journal for a period of seven days every second month to ensure you monitor your consumption of treat foods and frequency of dining out. It also allows you to reflect on your hunger scale throughout the day

to make sure you are still eating your largest meal at the start and smallest meal at the end of the day.

3. Cooking enough food every night so that you have plenty for lunch leftovers the following day. We don't have enough time to cook or prepare every single meal, so make things easy for yourself.

4. Eating your evening meal from a rice bowl or off a bread-and-butter plate.

5. Continuing to grocery shop once per week to avoid impulse buying and to ensure you always plan your meals for the week.

6. Revisiting your exercise routine every quarter to ensure you are not doing the same thing day in, day out. You should change what you are doing so that you continue to enjoy your exercise routine and challenge your body with a new stimulus.

7. Continuing to move! It doesn't matter what you do as long as it's regular and part of your daily routine. A wearable device that tracks your activity is a great way to keep an eye on it.

8. Going to bed at the same time and waking up at the same time each day.

9. Keeping an ongoing to-do list so that you are always working on constructive and positive activities in your life.

What should you do if you fall pregnant on your weight-loss journey?

As I've said, obesity is one of the biggest causes of infertility. Therefore, a common reason for women to lose weight is so they can fall pregnant. In some instances, it only takes a small weight loss of just a couple of kilograms for this to happen. But not everyone is this lucky, and it might require a much greater weight loss (for example, 10 kilograms or 20 kilograms). Also, there can be myriad reasons for infertility, not just your weight. It is very common for women hoping to fall pregnant to do so at some point along their IWL journey before they reach their goal set point. This is a very happy moment for those who have been trying to conceive for many years and it is a result of the body working more efficiently. But in saying all of this, it is much better to practise methods of contraception until you reach your goal set point before then trying to conceive. This will give you the best chance of a lifetime of not having to worry about your weight following the birth of your child or children.

If you do happen to fall pregnant on your IWL journey, further weight loss is *not* advised. At this time, you should immediately cease any further attempt to lose weight. In fact, you and your baby need extra food and nutrition (about one and a third times more) during the time of pregnancy. You will continue with the IWL plan, but you must put a halt on any further weight loss.

What should you do if you are overweight and you fall pregnant?

One in two women start their pregnancy journey above a healthy weight. Carrying extra weight at conception can increase your risk of complications during pregnancy such as high blood pressure, gestational diabetes, miscarriage and caesarean delivery. It can also be associated with complications for your baby including large birth weight, stillbirth and birth defects. Implementing methods of contraception to ensure you hit your new goal set point before falling pregnant will also significantly reduce the chances of your baby having weight problems throughout childhood and adolescence – a path that everyone wants to avoid for their children.

In an ideal world what I strongly encourage is, if you have the time, keep implementing methods of contraception to ensure you hit your new goal set point before falling pregnant. This is, of course, only relevant if your fertility will not decline to the point of being unfeasible before you hit that weight. What I mean by this is whether the biological clock is still on your side. To find out more about your situation you should talk to your general practitioner.

If you do fall pregnant while still carrying excess weight, don't panic. This is not the time to continue losing weight. You can, however, further reduce complications relating to pregnancy if you continue to implement all the principles of the IWL plan, without a weight-loss focus. This will see you making the switch to a healthier lifestyle that incorporates better food choices, better sleep and more exercise (at least 150 minutes of moderate-intensity exercise per week – more on this later).

How much weight gain is expected during pregnancy?

Irrespective of your weight when you fall pregnant, it is healthy to put on weight as a normal part of pregnancy. Don't panic when you start to see the scales change – you're growing a person! The only alarm will be if your husband puts on weight too. The term 'baby weight' can apply as much to men as to women. Whether it be attributed to less sleep, less time, more stress, those unhealthy cravings your partner might experience or an increase in portion sizes to coincide with your increase in appetite, they tend to put on a little during the time you're growing your baby and it's something to be mindful of. This is a time when your partner should be continuing with all aspects of the IWL plan while you put a hold on the weight-loss focus.

If you were overweight at the time of conception (as clinically diagnosed by BMI 25 kg/m² or above), a weight gain of 9 kilograms over the gestation period is healthy and expected. And of course, if you are pregnant with twins, this will be approximately double – a 20 kilogram weight gain over the gestation period.

If you fall pregnant in a healthy weight range, you can expect an even greater weight gain during pregnancy of approximately 12.5 kilograms, with most of this weight being gained after 20 weeks. By the time you reach your due date, more than a third of your extra weight will come from your baby (approximately 3.3 kilograms), the placenta (0.7 kilograms) and amniotic fluid (0.8 kilograms). But your body also changes to help grow and nourish your baby, which accounts for the other two-thirds of expected weight gain. You will see an increase in breast size, increased blood volume, extra body fluid, a bigger uterus, and 4 kilograms of fat to give you energy supplies for breastfeeding.

The moral of the story is that if you keep up your daily exercise and make healthy food choices, it doesn't matter what you gain while pregnant. By making sensible decisions about what you put into your body and how you treat it, you can let your incredible body look after itself. After you have safely delivered a healthy bub and recovered, you can then focus on implementing the weight-loss months of the IWL program again.

Tina had recently turned 30 when I first saw her. She reported that her weight had gone up by 6 kilograms over the past three years since taking on a more senior role in a bank and that she now weighed 72 kilograms, which was 10 kilograms above what she wanted to be. Tina and her husband had been trying for a baby for the past two years but had not changed her lifestyle during this time, using the common excuse that she had very little time for herself, largely due to her job. Thankfully Tina did not go and start a diet, despite her best friend's well-intended advice. Instead, we got her started on the IWL plan. She struggled at first to make time for exercise. In fact, for the first two months, all she did was find excuses: she investigated the cost of in-vitro fertilisation (IVF), and she continued with her sedentary lifestyle and poor food choices. However, after realising that IVF wasn't the answer and that change was necessary, she started slowly. One habit formed into another, and before she knew it she was looking for all sorts of opportunities to exercise. She began taking the stairs at work and imposed a ban on herself from using the lift. She then started taking public transport instead of driving to work. Not long after, Tina began a structured exercise routine and started playing soccer with her work colleagues at lunchtimes, most weekdays. Exercise became a way of life, and she enjoyed it. She had to carefully monitor her weight during the weight-maintenance periods to ensure it didn't continue going down. This was her biggest challenge after discovering her new love for sport. She continued to implement the six principles of the IWL plan and at the end of six months – and 5.5 kilograms lighter – Tina fell pregnant. She wanted to continue losing weight because she hadn't reached her goal weight loss, but I strongly advised that this would not be possible and would be dangerous to the health of her baby. After the healthy delivery of her child, she would then be able to implement the weight-loss months of the IWL plan to work towards the initial goal set point she aimed for.

How can you control your weight during pregnancy?

During pregnancy, you continue with all the principles of the IWL plan without a focus on weight loss – that is, every month of the IWL plan becomes a weight-maintenance month. (The same advice applies if you reach your goal weight loss on the IWL plan – you don't just stop the plan. More on this later.) The plan becomes a way of life and you must continue to implement all principles of the IWL plan while taking a focus off further weight loss. This means exercise is particularly important during pregnancy in order to prevent excessive weight gain. Despite what you might think, it is possible for you to exercise right up until the time of delivery (I will discuss this in greater detail in Chapter 10). The only difference is your food intake may increase to one and a third times your current intake on the IWL plan. You must continue eating all the foods outlined in the plan and you must ensure you do not deprive yourself of food. If you're hungry, you must eat! This will allow your body and your baby to thrive with the nutrition they need.

Why is every pregnancy different in terms of weight gain?

Your body will respond differently with every pregnancy, and you may experience varying degrees of weight gain with each one. This will largely depend on the weight you were before each pregnancy as well as how you manage your eating habits, sleep and activity during each one. Pregnancy can result in emotional turmoil, which subsequently leads to comfort eating or overeating. It can also result in different food cravings such as the hot chips you find yourself ordering for lunch every day or the chocolate bar you chow down to give yourself the afternoon pick-up. The same principles of the IWL plan always apply, and they will help ensure you gain a healthy amount of weight during pregnancy and provide the necessary nutrition that your baby needs for growth and development. Ensure you eat regularly to prevent excessive hunger and always reach for nature first to avoid giving in to your cravings.

Returning to pre-pregnancy weight

Most of the 9–12.5 kilogram weight increase that will occur during pregnancy will disappear in the first six months following the delivery of your child, if you are following the principles of the IWL plan. If you are then planning a subsequent pregnancy and have returned to your pre-pregnancy weight – that is, the weight you were before falling pregnant – you can then re-implement the principles of the weight-loss months of the IWL plan. Consider the case study, Tina. She had lost 5.5 kilograms of her 10 kilogram goal weight loss before falling pregnant. During her pregnancy, and for six months post-delivery, Tina continued to implement all the principles of the IWL plan as if she were following the weight-maintenance months. When she returned to her pre-pregnancy weight, five months after the delivery of her first child, she then kicked back into gear with the weight-loss months of the plan. Tina went on to lose the extra 4 kilograms of weight over the next five months (her body was very stubborn when she first re-initiated the weight-loss months, so it took her longer than she hoped), taking her cumulative weight-loss total to 9.5 kilograms. She fell pregnant for a second time, two years after giving birth to her first child, and she was nearly 10 kilograms lighter than when I first met her. She continued to implement the six principles of the IWL plan as a way of life and had two healthy children. This could have been very different if Tina had gone on a diet. Not only could she be 10 kilograms heavier, but she would also have had a life-long struggle with her weight and so too might her kids.

Why is weight loss after the second or third baby harder than the first?

Dropping those post-delivery kilos can be tough and each time different to the one before. However, the fact you might find it harder getting back to your pre-pregnancy weight after the second, third or subsequent babies has nothing to do with your body's physiology; it's to do with the fact that caring for two little ones is more challenging than one. This becomes even more relevant the more children you have. Your newborn will have completely different requirements to a five-year-old and consequently you will find you have less time for yourself as you devote more time to them. You often neglect your health, falling down the bottom of the priority list when it comes to things to do – you neglect exercise, you see a reduction in your sleep quality and quantity, and you fail to devote time to meal planning and preparation.

But the good news is that your body is still thriving and hasn't slowed down. If you give your body the chance and start to follow the principles of the IWL plan, you can get back to the weight you've always dreamt of. The IWL plan will help you overcome these common struggles so that you embed health into your day-to-day life. You must move away from the common identity excuse of not having enough time. Let's take exercise, for example. You don't need to go to the gym if you incorporate exercise into your daily routine – even if it means just pushing the pram around the neighbourhood or around the park while your other little ones play on the equipment. It might also mean attending a gym that offers childcare services while you work out. When it comes to food preparation, you need to ensure you or your partner attend to the weekly grocery shopping. And if that doesn't work, have your weekly groceries delivered. This option is also likely to reduce the risk of any baby or toddler tantrums in the supermarket.

What about IVF?

There is no question that obesity is now a leading cause of infertility. It's also a reason why more people are turning to IVF – a procedure used to overcome infertility by which an egg and sperm are joined together outside the body in a laboratory before then being transplanted into a woman's uterus to increase the chance of pregnancy occurring. IVF is invasive and requires hormone injections, not to mention the huge cost of thousands of dollars. And there's no guarantee it will work; only one in three women will succeed and have a baby on their first cycle of IVF, but your chance of success will decrease if you're older than 35 and/or carrying extra weight, highlighting the importance of losing weight before undergoing the procedure to increase your chance of success, if you are set on going down the route of IVF.

It is also important to stress that many women go through IVF for medical reasons, not because they're overweight. Such medical conditions include blocked or damaged fallopian tubes, uterine fibroids, endometriosis, problems with ovulation, male infertility or unexplained infertility. Regardless of whether you are successful, there are risks and unpleasant side effects associated with IVF. This is due to the invasive nature of the procedures and the fertility medications you're required to take. You may experience nausea, vomiting, bleeding, stomach pains and bloating, as well as weight gain from the hormone injections. Weight gain is especially common if the drugs used to induce ovulation cause your ovaries to become overstimulated – a condition known as ovulation hyperstimulation syndrome, which affects about 5 per cent of women.

If you do experience weight gain from the procedure, reflect and acknowledge that you've been through a huge ordeal and be kind to yourself. Allow your body to recover from what it has been through and go through the motions of the IWL 'wash-out' month – a key part of success for anyone starting on the IWL plan.

Age and pregnancy

The number of women having babies later in life – in their 30s and 40s – and close to the age of menopause is increasing. Until women have reached what is known as the post-menopausal stage, they can still fall pregnant. This can make weight loss more challenging post-delivery of your baby, but only if you continue with poor lifestyle habits, especially as we tend to become less active with age. By following the principles of the IWL plan, you will be able to lose the weight just as effectively as your counterpart 10 years younger.

The struggle with menopause

I have just discussed specifics relating to pregnancy, but another big challenge in life for women relates to menopause. This starts with perimenopause, otherwise known as transition to menopause, and begins a few years before menopause (typically lasting around four years). For most, it will start in their 40s. This marks the time when the ovaries start making less estrogen, and ends when a woman has gone 12 months without having her period. Symptoms are many and varied and can include irregular periods, hot flushes, fatigue, tender breasts, night sweats, vaginal dryness, difficulty sleeping, changes in mood and lower libido. Typically, women reach menopause, which marks the end of menstruation in a woman's life, between the ages of 45 and 55 but it can happen much earlier or as late as 60. Considering the average life expectancy of women in developed countries is 81 years, women will spend about 40 per cent of their life in post-menopause – so it's important to implement the principles of the IWL plan to prevent the common weight gain that accompanies menopause.

Why does weight gain happen during menopause?

Many of my patients often blame their weight gain on menopause. Yes, the hormonal changes of menopause – characterised by the progressive decline of endogenous estrogen levels – might make certain areas such as your stomach, hips and thighs more prone to weight gain, but hormonal changes aren't the reason. The weight gain is a by-product of ageing, and this is the time you must work hardest at your health. As we age, our body stops working as efficiently as it did before – much like an old car. Muscle mass starts to decrease with age – a fancy term known as 'sarcopenia' – and fat begins to increase. And because muscle mass is one of the determining factors of how fast your metabolism will run, when your muscle mass decreases, your body starts to burn fewer calories at rest, consequently making it more challenging to maintain your weight. As we age, we tend to continue with our same food habits and fail to increase our activity – aches and pains can make some people actively decrease theirs. This lack of compensation for the ageing process then results in a change in body composition and resulting weight gain.

The decline in estrogen and progesterone

Coupled with weight gain relating to the ageing process, menopause can also put you at risk of other health concerns such as heart disease, stroke and osteoporosis (weak or brittle bones). Following menopause your ovaries make very little of the hormones estrogen and progesterone. Estrogen helps to keep your blood vessels dilated – relaxed and open – which helps keep your cholesterol level down, so without it your bad cholesterol (known as low-density lipoprotein (LDL)-cholesterol) starts to build up in your arteries. This can increase your risk of heart disease and stroke. Furthermore, having less estrogen results in a loss of bone mass, putting you at risk of the disease osteoporosis, which makes your bones more prone to fractures.

How do you prevent weight gain during menopause?

Everything I have just told you is not to say you can't overcome any of these risks. You most definitely can, but it is a time of your life when you need to work harder on your health, with a specific focus on increasing your physical activity. If you focus on implementing everything articulated in this book – the six principles of the IWL plan – you will help prevent associated health risks and weight gain associated with this stage of life. There are many benefits in also talking to those who have already been through menopause, to learn from their experiences and to implement some of their tips. You can do this in the 'Interval Weight Loss Community' Facebook group where there are people at all stages of life implementing or who have already succeeded on the IWL plan.

What if you have already gone through menopause?

The good news is you can still overcome the health risks associated with menopause and reverse the weight you put on during menopause. And all of this is achieved by following the IWL plan. The first few months will be the hardest, because it is a time of your life when the body is most resistant to change. Exercise plays a vital role and you must start to include regular activity in your lifestyle. Focus on making one small change at a time, because these will turn into big changes and eventually become a way of life.

What about hormone replacement therapy?

The current role of hormone replacement therapy (HRT) is for relief of symptoms associated with menopause. It is important to ask your doctor if HRT is appropriate for you. If required, it should only be prescribed at the lowest effective dose and for the shortest duration required for the control of bothersome menopausal symptoms. It will not influence your weight change throughout menopause.

CHAPTER 16

YOUR TASKS

Throughout the book I have left you with specific tasks to complete. Here is a summary of them, and it is your job to make sure you have completed each one before kickstarting the IWL plan.

Chapter 1: Write down on a palm card the following quote: 'If you always do what you've always done, you'll always get what you've always got.'

Chapter 2: Take ownership of your actions by writing down all your identity excuses and rephrasing them into identity-accountability statements. Put them on palm cards and stick them throughout your home or in a place that is highly visible.

Chapter 3: Write a letter to yourself about what success means to you. It might just be a sentence devoting a commitment to yourself that you wish to become a better mum, to shape a better future for your children or to lead a healthier life. It should include three motivations/goals. These goals should be written down using the template provided in the book; each goal should have a range and must specify what new habit you will form, to replace the old with the new.

Chapter 4: Write down the six principles of the IWL plan, or go to the Interval Weight Loss website and sign up for the online program for your step-by-step guide to the six principles.

Chapter 5: Calculate your current and goal set point and record the values on a palm card.

Chapter 6: Purchase a set of scales. I suggest going to your local sports store to explore your options. Your will also need a weight tracker, available from the online program or you can download a template from the IWL website.

Chapter 7: Start recording in your phone every time you have a treat. At the end of the week tally them up and slowly work towards reducing their frequency over time. This might also become one of your goals that you set. For example:

Goal: Reduce frequency of chocolate bar consumption to 1–3 days per week.

New Behaviour: Increase consumption of nuts and seeds to 4–6 days per week.

Secondly, start recording how much you spend each day on food. Sit down with your partner or a friend and tally it up at the end of each week. You might even use this opportunity to catch up socially and go out for your weekly dining-out meal.

Chapter 8: Write down or photocopy the list of foods to include on the IWL plan, as well as the list of foods you can snack on between breakfast, lunch and dinner.

Chapter 9: Buy yourself a set of chopsticks or a teaspoon.

Chapter 10: Monitor your current activity level using a wearable device. If you don't have a wearable device, it is well worth the investment and you will find some great deals if you shop around. Add structured activity to your calendar (a month's worth) and ensure you alternate the days so that non-body weight bearing exercise appears between days of body weight bearing exercise. You don't have to include structured exercise every day (perhaps every second day to start) but you need to gradually build it up over the month.

Chapter 11: Write your own to-do list and keep it in a place that is highly visible and handy so you can continually update it. Whenever something pops in your head that needs to be actioned, write it on this list. You can use the template in the book.

Ongoing task

I want you to regularly reflect on the goals you set, as per the task in Chapter 3. Have you made any progress on your goals? If not, this is not a problem but just a reminder of what you are trying to achieve and it may need some adjustment. I want you to add one extra goal to your letter and palm card every 66 days. Remember, this is the time it takes to form a new habit.

CHAPTER 17

CASE STUDIES

These are real-life case studies of people who are currently part of the IWL community and following the IWL plan. Their names have been changed to maintain anonymity.

CASE STUDY 1: LAURA

Laura first reached out to me after the launch of my second book – *Interval Weight Loss For Life*. Like most people following the IWL plan, she was very keen to get into the program and was at the point, after dieting her whole life, of never wanting to diet again. But before getting started, she was struggling to get over one basic first step – how much to eat at each meal time. Laura understood that she was supposed to have more at breakfast and less at dinner but still wanted to be prescribed exact portions and serving sizes. This had been engrained into her psyche from a lifetime of dieting and it was going to take some time to help her get over this barrier.

Laura: I have a question about evening meals. The books talk about eating a much smaller dinner than what people are used to. Should you ignore hunger at night, particularly when you first start the IWL program?

I explained to Laura that if she focused on more food at the start of the day, she would find that, over time, her hunger signals would change and she would become less hungry in the evening, and hence the smaller portion would be sufficient. I emphasised that this wouldn't happen overnight and that it was imperative that breakfast and lunch become far more important meals (from a portion perspective) than dinner. I also encouraged her to go back and re-read the books to help better instil the principles of the IWL plan.

Laura: I have re-read the books, thanks. I would really like to do the plan but am still struggling with how much food to eat. I am the 'typical' case talked about in the books: hungriest in the afternoon/evenings and have been on literal starvation diets over the last few years. Consequently, I am often hungry and hate it, so I eat! I am still feeling a bit lost with how to implement this into my life.

I gave Laura one goal – to simply implement the change of big to small meals throughout the day and to not worry about how much she was serving up, if it was based on the foods outlined in the IWL plan.

Her case is typical of many patients I have seen and many of those in the community following the IWL plan. It may also resonate with you, and if it does, you too need to adopt the same mindset as Laura. A mindset based on a lifetime of dieting does not change overnight, but it does change! Laura, like many other people in the IWL community, is a wonderful example of such success.

Laura: I have decided to forget about trying to lose weight for a while. My weight gain over the years is 100 per cent the result of having the all-or-nothing approach to diet and exercise. For the past 30-ish years I have either been putting on weight or losing it, with the losing part getting harder and harder as the years have gone on. I have either been on a diet or planning my next diet with the planning diet phase including lots of overeating of the foods I am 'never going to eat again' because, of course, this next diet will be the one that works and stops me from eating all the foods that I believe have made me gain weight.

After reading both of the IWL books, I have now realised that when I first started I got straight into approaching it exactly like I have with all my 'next diet phases', and in my first month of planned weight loss I ended up obsessing over food and would often be hungry all the time again, which eventually ended with the usual over-eating, self-loathing, feelings-of-failure phase, injuring myself from over-exercising, obsessing over the scales, weighing myself every day, experiencing the usual happiness that comes with any loss and misery/self-loathing that comes with any gain, even 100 grams!

So, after week two I decided to stop the weight-loss month, and I am not even sure when I will start one again. Instead I am working on changing my habits and my mindset, one step at a time. These three things are where I am putting my energy and focus:

1. *I am now diligently exercising for an hour, six days a week, doing something I really enjoy. I am doing it because it has a huge positive influence on both my mental and physical health.*

2. *I remind myself daily that my weight is the natural response to the years of dieting, it is not because I am lazy or lacking will-power, and being overweight does not define me.*

3. *I am paying serious attention to the food I eat, but in a completely different way. I eat when I am hungry, I eat what I feel like eating (I have even gone back to enjoying meals out with my friends and family instead of turning everything down out of fear of not wanting to have a 'food disaster'!), and I do*

my best to stop when I am 80 per cent full (this one is really hard as I am so used to under- and overeating).

4. *I haven't lost any weight but guess what, I haven't put any on either. And for now, that is more than enough. I have NEVER been in a position of eating 'freely' and not gaining weight. I am starting to trust my appetite instead of fearing it, it's a good feeling!*

Laura introduced the following three things when first starting off and that helped her overcome her initial barriers to the plan.

1. Forget about portion sizes and focus on simply eating more at the start of the day and less at the end of the day.

This allowed her to start appreciating how her appetite signalling worked in the body and to adjust portion sizes according to what her body was demanding. For those who need more guidance I suggest sticking to my very broad guide: breakfast will be a portion size equivalent to three hand fists, lunch will be approximately two hand fists, and the evening meal will be approximately one hand fist. This is just to kickstart you on the IWL plan and then you can make the necessary alterations. For example, some people will need four hand fists of food (or more) at breakfast, three at lunch and two at dinner, while other people may need less. As long as you are following the funnel plan of big to small throughout the day, you are on track and you will start to appreciate how the appetite signalling works in your body, paying particular attention to the hunger scale provided in this book.

2. Take the focus off body weight.

Laura focused on changes in her health rather than a change on the scales. As weekly weighing (but no more than this) is a crucial part of IWL, she still weighed herself but reflected on how she felt both physically and mentally from the new habits she was forming.

3. Do not cut out any foods.

Putting certain foods in the 'forbidden' pile is destined for disaster. Learning that she could enjoy all foods on the IWL plan meant that she was able to remove the fear from certain foods and regain a healthy relationship with foods she had previously forbidden.

For many people, just like Laura, the dieting mentality is the hardest thing to shift. Many of you are very good at instigating dietary changes, because you have often done it thousands of times before. Yes, the IWL plan requires you to weigh yourself each week but you must take the goal away from weight loss. Having weight loss as the ultimate, single goal can be completely detrimental to what you are achieving, which is sustained life-long changes. Our modern society supports the paradigm whereby weight loss = success, and weight gain = failure. You will only end up measuring your entire self-worth by how much you weigh on the scales, and this is what you want to prevent.

CASE STUDY 2: JANE

Millions of people have been brainwashed by the diet industry with that all-too-familiar message: to lose weight you must eat less and move more. The way you do that is to count calories and that if you do the maths right – that is, consume fewer calories than you burn each day – the results will show. People then obsessively track every meal they consume in one of these fancy and costly apps, only to be bemused and disheartened when they see the result on the scales.

Jane's experience is a case study that is typical of so many people.

I first met Jane 10 years ago. She had been a serial dieter all her life and tried every diet you could imagine. Some of them I hadn't even heard of. I knew this was going to be a tough challenge, to successfully free her of the dieting mindset that was ingrained in her. She was also going through menopause and was attributing her recent weight gain to this change in her life.

After telling her how to implement the Interval Weight Loss plan, I asked her to report back in two months. This allowed her time to complete a one-month wash-out, as well as a one-month weight-loss month, presuming her weight was not still increasing at the end of the wash-out. This was because she had recently come off a 'eat right for your blood-type' diet and wasn't sure if she had regained all the weight she lost.

Jane: I have done what you prescribed; I completed a wash-out for a month and my weight was stable at the end of the four weeks at 89 kilograms. I then kicked off a weight-loss month. After an initial loss in the first couple of weeks – 0.3 kilograms in the first week and 0.8 kilograms in the second week – I was excited by what I had seen. However, my weight has not budged in the last couple of weeks and I fear I've done something wrong. I really did everything you're supposed to do. I logged everything in an excel spreadsheet and used a calorie-counting platform to work out the exact calories I was putting in my body. I cut out all the high-fat and processed food, and I'm even doing an hour of exercise every day, but the weight still isn't going down. I feel tired and moody and need help!

Many of you will be familiar with Jane's situation. You would have logged everything you ate, gave up all the sweets, and even been diligent with your gym attendance. You may have seen a weight change on the scales but at some point this would have plateaued, and you would have regained all the weight you lost.

Sadly, Jane didn't have a good grasp of the Interval Weight Loss plan. She had failed to understand several fundamental aspects of the plan. First, she was calorie counting. You will know now from reading this book that calorie counting is a waste of time; it is crude and often misleading. Calculating the calorie content of food is far more complex than what the precise numbers of food packets might have you suggest. In fact, those numbers you see in apps or on food packets have a 20 per cent error rate, and on processed frozen foods it can be much higher. Furthermore, two items of food with identical calories may be digested in very different ways, again making the calorie label on the food redundant. For example, 20 per cent of the calories in nuts are not absorbed whereas most of the calories from a slice of pizza are.

Second, she had adopted the all-or-nothing approach to weight loss. She had cut out all the foods she had been led to believe were fattening and she had signed up to a three-month gym membership so she could go to the gym every day, even though she knew that this was not sustainable with juggling her children's commitments and her current financial situation.

A lifetime of dieting meant that Jane's body was quickly able to combat the stress she had imposed and had reacted by preventing further weight loss. This was only going to continue if she continued with this approach. We went through the principles of the IWL plan again. I advised Jane to make the following three simple changes and to not worry about anything else.

1. Abolish the idea of calorie counting and instead write food consumption in a journal.

This task meant that she no longer had to obsess over the number of calories she was eating in the course of the day. Instead, she was given the simple task of highlighting when she would eat a treat food or a takeaway/dining-out meal.

2. Track incidental activity on a wearable device.

This meant that Jane no longer had to go to the gym every day. Of course, Jane still went when she could, because she enjoyed a lot of the classes and had just paid for a three-month membership, but this simple task of tracking her incidental activity brought to her attention how sedentary she was. This allowed her to move her mindset away from the need for structured activity and instead actively think about ways to increase her incidental activity towards a minimum of 10,000 steps per day.

3. Ensure at least one treat food per week and one takeaway meal per week.
This resulted in a huge psychological shift in her mindset. Jane realised that she could still eat her favourite foods, that no foods were forbidden and that she would still get the result she was after on the scales.

After two months of successfully implementing these changes and not focusing on weight loss, Jane started to have some big wins. These small changes she had put into place led to much bigger changes, and over time she began to develop more and more positive habits. Over the course of four years, Jane lost 40 kilograms and has kept it off, but it wasn't an easy start and it may not be for you either, if you relate to her situation.

CASE STUDY 3: PENNY

I have seen patients with obesity from all walks of life, but the majority of those struggling with their weight have many commonalities. The first one relates to how many diets they have attempted and the other relates to how many people end up with an eating disorder from a lifetime of dieting.

Penny ticked each of these boxes. She had dieted extensively from the age of 11.

Penny: I'm reading your books and they make great sense to me. I was put on my first diet at the age of 11 by ballet teachers and developed a binge-eating disorder and obesity. I stopped dieting years ago but am still in recovery. I am still quite overweight and would like to lose it. I haven't weighed myself for years because I always become very obsessive and it's no good for me.

We agreed that the best way for Penny to address her concern with weighing was to first start with a wash-out month without weighing and then start weekly weighing (and waist-circumference measures) after a month of introducing all the principles in the IWL plan. Understandably, considering her fear of weighing and her history with a binge-eating disorder, she asked a friend or, when possible, her therapist, to support her around the required weekly weighing component of the IWL plan. Her homework was also to re-read the books, because it was going to take some time to unlearn all the confusing and incorrect information that Penny had been told over the years.

Positive changes became evident immediately. Aside from her weight loss, Penny's greatest success was that she managed to avoid the big binges that previous attempts to lose weight had triggered.

Penny introduced the following three things when first starting on the IWL plan.

1. Implement a wash-out period without monitoring weight.
This allowed Penny to introduce all the foods outlined in the plan without worrying about fluctuations in her body weight due to changes in the water content in the body. Previously, seeing an increase on the scales would trigger a binge-eating episode.

2. After the wash-out period, perform the weekly weigh-ins with a close friend or therapist.
This was the extra support that Penny needed on each weekly weigh-in.

3. Have IWL-approved snacks readily available to prevent long periods of not eating and subsequent binges of heavily processed foods.

This allowed Penny to retrain her brain away from her dependence on addictive foods such as chocolate and cake. She learnt to prevent hunger setting in by snacking frequently and would get the same pleasure response in the brain from nature's treats. When food shopping, she would go to the supermarket after eating and go to the checkout that was devoid of chocolates (believe it or not, there is one in every big supermarket chain).

Penny has lost some weight, but most importantly has restored a healthy relationship with food and regained control over her health both physically and mentally. She is in remission from her eating disorder and continues to lose weight as per the principles of the IWL plan.

CASE STUDY 4: LORNELLE

It's clearly established that people who are overweight suffer from a higher chance of infertility, so as you can imagine many of my patients want to lose weight so they can fall pregnant. Thankfully, these patients hadn't signed up to the latest diet that would have seen them lose weight and potentially fall pregnant, and then end up heavier down the track. Some had tried in-vitro fertilisation (IVF) treatment without any luck. For many, IVF was unattainable due to the high cost. In any case, a woman's weight can affect her success rate with IVF.

But the good news is, once you start to lose weight on the IWL plan, you increase your chance of ovulating normally, avoiding the need for fertility treatment. Weight loss will also decrease the risk of complications during pregnancy not only for you, but also for your baby.

Lornelle was a patient of mine seven years ago. She had been trying to fall pregnant for over three years before I met her. She had even tried IVF with no success. She had a busy corporate job and worked long hours, and after I explained to her the IWL plan, she accepted that her biggest challenge would be to restore her work–life balance. She could still work long hours, but she needed to devote time throughout the day to her health. This meant scheduling frequent blocks in her calendar to not only ensure she would eat regularly, but also allow time for structured activity. In addition, it meant preparing for the week ahead on Saturday or Sunday, so that she had an adequately stocked fridge to avoid eating out all the time.

Her first two months were slow, but some positive habits began to form. She started weighing herself once weekly (this was a huge change from her previous habit of weighing herself at least twice a day); she managed to increase her incidental activity by walking whenever she could (she banned the lift altogether); she included some form of structured activity at lunch every day of the week (a minimum of one hour would be blocked off in her calendar to allow ample time to shower and change afterwards); and her frequency of eating out at lunch decreased to once per week because she and her husband were making extra at dinner and taking leftovers for lunch the following day. But, all these positive changes aside, she still struggled with one of the key principles of the IWL plan: to have her biggest meal at the start of the day. She also struggled to change her evening routine of having a bottle of wine with her husband each night. Consequently, her weight didn't shift, and she was getting frustrated.

We reflected on all the wonderful changes that she had made. The portion size of breakfast was an easier barrier to overcome, but alcohol was more challenging. We developed a plan to deal with the evening routine. To break this habit of drinking alcohol every night, she needed to replace it with a new habit. She and her husband developed a to-do list of things they wanted to achieve over the next 12 months. One of the biggest ones was to save a deposit for a house and they worked out how much they could save from a reduction in alcohol intake alone. They had already started to make huge savings from the reduction in food eaten out at lunch. This was to be their challenge over the month.

Every evening, instead of reaching for a bottle of wine, they would get out the laptop and open the spreadsheet that they were using to track their daily expenditure. Each would record what they had spent for the day and it was a gentle reminder of what they were trying to achieve. They also used the evening time to commence a new hobby, which was learning French for a trip they were planning the following year. This new activity became a habit and it replaced the habit of drinking a bottle of wine every night. They still enjoyed some alcohol but kept it for a night when they went out for their weekly dining-out meal.

After eight months of following the IWL plan and a 6 kilogram weight loss, Lornelle fell pregnant. She was elated, but of course wanted to keep losing weight. I strongly advised her not to, explaining that she could continue her weight-loss journey after the birth of her child.

Lornelle had a healthy weight gain (10 kilograms) during her pregnancy which she was able to quickly drop in the first six months after delivery. She then continued to lower her set point after the birth of her first child and before falling pregnant again, taking her total weight loss to 10 kilograms (from 79 kilograms to 69 kilograms). The biggest improvement she noticed in her health was her vitality and energy levels. She would look forward to exercising every day and felt she was much more productive at work despite working slightly fewer hours.

Over the course of seven years, Lornelle has had two children and lost 20 kilograms following the IWL plan. The whole time she continued to follow all six principles of the IWL plan but did not implement weight-loss months during her pregnancies. Every now and then, she and her husband still implement the spend challenge and record how much each is spending. They continue to drink alcohol because they enjoy it but they can happily say that they no longer drink what they used to.

In this instance, it is important to reiterate that fertility issues due to excess weight are not just limited to women. If your partner is carrying some excess weight, he may need to follow the IWL plan with you.

Lornelle attributed the following points to kickstarting her success on the IWL plan.

1. Block off time each day for structured activity.
This became routine and it also began to inspire her colleagues to do the same every day.

2. Make extra food each evening so it could be taken as leftovers for lunch the following day.
Not only did this result in saving loads of money, it also guaranteed Lornelle had a healthier and more delicious meal for lunch each day.

3. Record daily expenditure on food and beverages to raise awareness of where money is being spent.
Importantly, this addressed the daily habit of drinking alcohol and saw Lornelle participating in fun and productive activities with her husband each evening, instead of sitting around on the couch mindlessly eating and drinking.

CHAPTER 18

COMMONLY ASKED QUESTIONS

These are commonly asked questions posed by the Interval Weight Loss community, and some of them also appear in books one and two. This section is designed to be a comprehensive catalogue of common stumbling blocks when first starting off on the IWL plan. However, if you have a question that isn't covered here, I encourage you to get in touch through the 'Dr Nick Fuller's Interval Weight Loss' Facebook page or to email me via the Interval Weight Loss website. Please do not hesitate to reach out, because this will ensure you succeed on the IWL plan.

Where do I go for further help?

All the advice you need is in this book. You can also sign up to the IWL online program for additional support on your IWL journey The good news is that you do not need face-to-face contact to succeed on the IWL plan. This plan can be followed by anyone, from wherever they are located – rural, remote and overseas. You will most benefit when you read the book more than once, especially if you have a history of dieting. Re-reading the book will help you break the dieting mindset and help unlearn all the bad habits and wrong information you may have picked up over the years.

It is imperative that you closely follow the plan as articulated in this book.

Re-reading the book will also help instil the principles and core methodology of the IWL plan. It is designed to be an easy, understandable and fun read. The list of foods you need to stick to on the IWL plan should be written down and stuck on your fridge so that every time you are hungry you are reminded what to eat.

I have had a long career as a clinical researcher dealing face-to-face with patients and now I want to reach as many people as possible through my books and online. You can engage with me on social media and you can ask me a question via intervalweightloss.com.au.

Is the IWL plan for everyone?

I have had countless enquiries about whether the IWL plan can be followed by people of different ethnicities or with different eating patterns. Yes, absolutely yes! It can be followed by anyone. The IWL plan is an adaptive approach that can be tailored to your lifestyle. If you're a vegetarian, take the meat out. If you're allergic to salmon, don't make the salmon recipe. If you're coeliac, substitute with wholegrain carbohydrates that don't contain gluten.

Is the IWL plan suitable for those with diabetes and polycystic ovary syndrome (PCOS)?

Yes, it is most certainly suitable for those with diabetes – both type 1 and type 2, and gestational diabetes (diabetes during pregnancy) – and PCOS. If you have type 2 diabetes, weight loss will help prevent the disease from progressing further and in some instances may help you get rid of the disease altogether. It is also suitable for those with insulin resistance or pre-diabetes (the stage before type 2 diabetes), because the weight loss you can achieve will see your body working properly again and prevent the disease. PCOS is a very common hormonal disorder that affects a woman's ovaries during childbearing years. The IWL plan will help you lose weight if you have PCOS and just a small amount of weight loss can help regulate ovulation and periods.

Can I follow the IWL plan while pregnant?

Yes, you should follow the IWL plan during pregnancy, but you must *not* lose any weight. Weight gain is healthy and expected during pregnancy. You are growing a person! After delivering your baby, you will find that you naturally bounce back to your pre-pregnancy weight within the first six months of childbirth, and even if you don't, there is no cause for concern. The IWL plan will help you get back there.

Is the IWL plan suitable for those with food intolerances?

Yes, if there is a recipe that includes milk, for instance, and you are lactose intolerant, you will need to substitute it with a lactose-free alternative, such as lactose-free milk. Similarly, those with coeliac disease will need to eliminate foods containing gluten or find a replacement for ingredients or products containing gluten. If you are diagnosed with lactose intolerance or coeliac disease and are still unsure which ingredients are suitable substitutes, please make contact through the Facebook page for some suggestions.

Is the IWL plan suitable for vegans or vegetarians?

Yes, most certainly. Again, simply substitute any meat or animal products with suitable alternatives. For example, meat with tofu, or chicken with beans. Refer to Chapter 8 for a key list of nutrients to be mindful of when following a vegan diet.

Can the IWL plan be followed by those with hypothyroidism or an under-active thyroid?

Yes, however it is vital to follow up with your general practitioner regarding your medication and dosage, and to ensure your thyroid function is regularly monitored with a blood test. Weight loss may improve your thyroid function and therefore your medication will need adjusting as you progress on the IWL plan.

Can the IWL plan be followed by those on medications for depression or other mental disorders?

Yes, but you should follow up with your general practitioner if you suspect weight gain due to the medication/s you are taking. There is a greater availability of approved medications for treatment of depression and mental disorders nowadays that do not have a negative effect on body weight, and these may be applicable to your condition.

Is the IWL plan suitable for those with cancer or in remission from cancer?

Yes. More and more cancers are being linked to obesity, so eating foods such as wholegrain carbohydrates, fruits and vegetables can only help. Please be aware, of course, that if you have cancer you will still need treatment – the IWL plan does *not* cure cancer.

Can I include wholegrain carbs if I am diagnosed with coeliac disease?

Yes, definitely. If you are diagnosed with coeliac disease, you need to avoid grains containing gluten such as wheat, rye and barley. Suitable gluten-free grains that are also rich in fibre include rice, quinoa, millet and amaranth and you should include plenty of them (see a full list of suitable wholegrains to include in your IWL plan in Chapter 8). There are also many foods that are naturally gluten-free – fruits, vegetables, dairy, meat, fish, nuts and eggs, to name a few. To get tested for coeliac disease, your GP may send you for a blood test in the first instance, but to confirm the result they will need to send you for an endoscopy – a specialised test where they check the lining of your intestine to see if it is functioning properly.

Can I substitute dishes/recipes with my own favourites?

Yes, absolutely. The daily meal and monthly plans are just a guide. This book is not intended to be a cookbook but rather give you some good ideas on what you can make, how easy it can be to cook using just a few ingredients, and to show you ingredients you should use as the foundations for all recipes. Remember, when following the IWL plan you don't need to rely on meal plans, count calories or weigh out portions of each ingredient. You can put any of your favourite recipes into the weekly food plan; you may just have to make some alterations to ensure they are based on the core principles of the IWL plan. Remember the following.

- Cook with raw ingredients.
- Cook with olive or canola oil only (preferably extra-virgin or cold-pressed).
- Include plenty of vegetables or salad vegetables with each recipe (including with pasta-based meals).
- Ensure you include a source of fat, protein and wholegrain carbohydrate with each recipe to ensure your daily meal plan is nutritionally balanced and includes all the core food groups at each meal.

You can sign up to a free weekly IWL recipe at the Interval Weight Loss website for more ideas.

How do I know how much to eat?

Intentionally, there is very little in my books and meal plans about exact quantities to eat. This is because it is *not a diet* and you will not succeed if you rely on a set 28-day plan, eight- or 12-week program, or similar.

We all need guidance, but you must learn how much to eat at each meal by listening to your body signals and by ensuring that you eat a lot at the start of the day and very little at the end of the day. For most, this will mean completely switching around the structure of your current food intake. When I mention oats for breakfast, load up your bowl on the first few occasions because breakfast is the most important meal of the day and should be the biggest (but you can split it up into two smaller breakfasts – one before work and one when you arrive at work). If you can't get through the portion or feel uncomfortably full at the end of the meal you have eaten too much, and you need to reduce the quantity the next day until you master it. This is because everyone needs a different intake; males will usually need more than females (sometimes one and a half times the intake) because they have a larger body mass.

The same applies to dinner. If a recipe specifies how many it serves, this is a guide that will enable you to make an appropriate amount to factor in leftovers for the next day's lunch. How much you cook depends on which meal you are using the recipe for. As per the IWL plan, you will serve up more at lunch than you would at dinner.

As a general rule of thumb, when you are first starting out on the IWL plan, and to give you something to work with as a guide, breakfast will be a portion size that is equivalent to three closed fists, lunch will be approximately two closed fists, and the evening meal will be approximately one closed fist. (Remember, these guides exclude vegetables, so you can load up as many vegetables and as much salad as you like at each meal.) Your food requirements will increase during pregnancy (particularly during the third trimester) and when breastfeeding – up to one and a third times the food you typically eat – and this is fine and encouraged.

Another great tool to use is the appetite scale provided in this book. This is particularly helpful when you are first starting the IWL plan to continually assess how hungry you are before and after each meal. You need to record this before and after each meal in a food journal and you should start this process in the wash-out period.

In summary, there are no exact portion sizes on the IWL plan. But you must remember that every meal must be balanced. Half the meal should be vegetables or salad, with a quarter being a wholegrain carbohydrate source such as a piece of bread or serve of rice, and a quarter being your protein source such as meat, fish or lentils.

How do I eat all the prescribed food when struggling with morning sickness?

Morning sickness is common during pregnancy, usually in the first trimester, and mostly due to changing levels of pregnancy hormones. It's vital to keep well hydrated, even if you can only manage small, frequent sips of fluid. Soups are another great way of keeping up your fluid intake to prevent dehydration. During this time, it is more appropriate to eat smaller, more regular meals. It is also advised to avoid any smells of foods that makes your nausea worse, and you may need to focus on including blander food. Aside from this, the same principles of the IWL plan apply.

What size should my evening meal be?

It should fit onto a bread-and-butter plate or a rice bowl. You can eat as many vegetables or as much salad as you like. If you are hungry after having this small portion for dinner you should wait 10 minutes before considering going back for a second portion. In this instance, you may need to start eating more food at the start of the day to ensure you are less hungry by the time dinner comes around. And don't forget your chopsticks!

What volume does a rice bowl hold?

A rice bowl is a small bowl used in Asian cuisine for rice. It's the perfect tool for measuring out your evening meal and should be approximately the size of your fist.

Is it bad to eat late at night?

It is not always practical to have an early dinner. Eat dinner when you can but make sure it is the smallest meal of the day. This is even more important when having your evening meal later in the evening because you are less likely to wake up feeling hungry if you overeat at night.

I never wake up hungry. What should I do?

It takes time for your hunger cues to change, and if you have been doing the same thing for years or decades – that is, skipping breakfast because you didn't feel hungry – your body's signals will not change overnight. Coffee can also mask your appetite, so make sure to have something with your morning coffee. If you have changed your meal orientation to ensure you are having your smallest meal at dinner you are well on the way to success and you will start to wake up feeling hungrier. Just give it time! This change is not going to happen overnight, but ride it out – it's worth it, I promise.

What should I eat during the maintenance period? Do I just eat the same way I've been eating during the weight-loss month but have more dinner?

You should structure your food intake in the same way during the maintenance periods as in the weight-loss months – largest meal at breakfast and smallest meal at dinner. You should not be eating more at dinner. The maintenance months allow you the flexibility to include more of those treat foods you love or to eat out more regularly. For a detailed explanation of how to adjust your eating plan in the weight-maintenance months refer to Chapter 14.

How much should I eat during pregnancy?

Your appetite will increase during the second and particularly third trimester of pregnancy. This is normal and you need to welcome this increase in appetite. It may mean you're eating one and a third times the quantity of food you typically eat on the IWL plan (this is fine and encouraged). Remember, you are growing another person and they are dependent on good nutrition to grow and develop. Always remember to *reach for nature first* and whenever you have cravings for junk, think about your health and that of your baby. Listen to your body's appetite signalling and feed it the fuel it needs. If you're still hungry after eating, have some more.

How much should I eat while breastfeeding?

Much like during pregnancy, your appetite will increase when breastfeeding and will only start to decrease when your baby starts to eat solids. Making breastmilk burns a lot of calories and you need extra food to meet these requirements. Again, just like when you're pregnant, you may be eating one and a third times the guide portions on the IWL plan, and this is perfectly fine. You need to listen to what your body is telling you – if you're hungry, you need to eat. Remember, the breastmilk you are producing is your baby's only fuel source, and the nutrition you take in will influence its food preferences later in life. Eat according to the IWL plan and, importantly, focus on a rich variety of foods.

What should I do if I gain weight after going on the Pill?

Weight gain from taking the oral contraceptive Pill is a common complaint. There can be many side effects from taking the Pill, including weight gain, mood instability, bleeding and decrease in sex drive. Most of the time the weight gain is transient (much like many of the unpleasant side effects from taking the Pill) and due to fluid retention – it should go away with time. The other good news is that research shows no effect on weight from taking the Pill. But in saying this, if you think your weight has been increasing due to the Pill, talk to your doctor, because there are many different options available and it is important to find one that works for you.

What should I do if my weight isn't going down during the weight-loss month?

The most important thing is to monitor the trend in your weight change over time. If you don't lose weight in a particular month, don't be disheartened; instead, focus on all the wins you have had and reflect on all the positive changes you are experiencing in your health, aside from weight loss.

If I don't lose any weight in a weight-loss month should I try another weight-loss month?

No, you must move on to your weight-maintenance month as per the IWL plan. This is very common when first starting off on the IWL plan, especially if you have recently been on a diet or have been on numerous diets in the past. Your body becomes very efficient at removing any stress associated with dieting and it may mean you have to follow the wash-out period for longer than you hoped. But you will still get there and you need to focus on the long-term picture.

If you know it's going to be a challenging month (for example, you might be caring for someone, have a lot of family commitments or it's Christmas time), this is also a well-advised time to embrace a weight-maintenance month. Sometimes, two or more weight-maintenance months in a row are required, and this is completely fine.

Is all sugar bad for you?

Since the 'sugar-free' and 'I Quit Sugar' movements became popular, there has been much confusion about what constitutes a sugar and the difference between various types of sugar. Added sugars and naturally occurring sugars are not the same thing. Many foods contain naturally occurring sugars and these foods are very good for us (for example, fruit and dairy). They are excellent sources of nutrition and important for our long-term health. Do not let someone convince you that because a food contains 'sugar' it is bad for you. They are wrong. Naturally occurring sugars, such as glucose, fructose, sucrose, lactose and maltose are good for us and not part of the obesity problem because they are contained in foods that are wholesome and nutritious.

Added sugars are the 'bad' sugars and you will find them predominantly in food products coming out of a packet, such as muesli bars, or in white refined carbs such as pastries, confectionary and sweets. As a rule of thumb, food in its natural form may contain sugars that are naturally occurring and good for us, and food coming out of a packet may contain added sugars that are bad for us. As has been reiterated throughout this book, there is no need to restrict any foods in their naturally occurring form.

Does sugar cause diabetes?

Sugar in foods does *not* cause diabetes. Type 1 diabetes is an auto-immune disease (there is no cure and it can't be prevented, people are often born with it) and type 2 diabetes is typically caused by carrying excess body weight, which consequently stops the body working as efficiently as it should. Gestational diabetes is a type of diabetes developed during pregnancy (closely aligned with type 2 diabetes) and typically goes away following the birth of your child.

However, if you do develop it, it is vital to manage it by following the principles of the IWL plan (without a focus on weight loss), which will reduce your possibility of pregnancy complications and risk to your newborn (large baby, miscarriage and stillbirth). It will also reduce your risk of gestational diabetes persisting post childbirth and resulting in type 2 diabetes.

Foods that contain *added* sugar and fat, such as pastries, chocolates, ice-cream or anything that is processed and coming out of a packet, are high in energy. If you regularly include a high intake of these foods, it is likely you will be eating too many calories and put on weight, and may down the track develop type 2 diabetes. However, sugar itself does not cause diabetes.

It is a perplexing field to navigate when wading through the supermarket, and there are more than 50 names for sugar. The most common ingredients to watch out for when looking for added sugars on labels include:

- brown sugar
- corn syrup
- fruit juice concentrates
- glucose solids
- high-fructose corn syrup
- invert sugar
- malt sugar
- molasses
- raw sugar
- sugar molecules ending in 'ose' (e.g. dextrose, glucose, sucrose, maltose, fructose).

Doesn't fruit have sugar and therefore need to be avoided?

Yes, fruit does contain sugar but these are naturally occurring sugars. These are nature's treats and should form part of your daily eating plan. You can eat as much fruit as you like, as long as it's not juiced or dried. Juicing means most of the goodness (the fibre) gets left behind in the juicer, and dried fruit has had the water stripped out of it, so it's very easy to overconsume. Fruit or other foods containing naturally occurring sugars do not cause diabetes or weight gain. No fruits will make you fat and you can eat all fruits on the IWL plan (yes, even bananas!).

If I buy skim or low-fat milk will it have added sugar?

Skim, no-fat or low-fat milk will not have added sugar. The only difference between full-fat and the low-fat or skim alternatives is that the fat is literally skimmed off the top of the milk. Skim or low-fat will have the same protein and calcium without the fat.

Some milks do have added sugar – such as almond milk, oat milk and other dairy alternatives. Read the label carefully.

Which milk is best?

Cow's milk is the richest source of calcium, protein and iodine. If you are looking for a dairy-free and lactose-free alternative to cow's milk, calcium-fortified soy milk is the next best option from a nutritional perspective. Rice milk and almond milk are low in protein. Tune in to my podcast with Dr Karl on 'white milk scams' – it's one of my favourite podcasts with Dr Karl to date. You will find all my podcasts with Dr Karl at the University of Sydney's 'Shirtloads of Science' page (shirtloadsofscience.libsyn. com) and on the Interval Weight Loss website.

Which yoghurt should I choose?

You do need to be a little careful with yoghurt. No-fat or low-fat yoghurt can have added sugar to make up for the loss of flavour incurred by removing the fat. Find one that says 'low fat' *and* 'no added sugar' on the label. This is typically natural yoghurt. The full-fat variety is fine too.

Is full-fat dairy okay?

Yes, it is. All that matters is that you include dairy every day – two to three serves per day. Research has clearly documented that those who include more dairy products in their daily eating plan have lower body weight, better heart health and are better able to manage their weight than those who don't include them. We don't know whether full-fat dairy is bad for our waistline, and until this question is answered through research, I would advise you to stick to skim dairy and base your dairy intake around milk and yoghurt products. It has the same nutrition – calcium and protein – as the full-fat variety with half the calories. You can buy no-fat and low-fat yoghurt without added sugar or you can opt for plain, natural yoghurt and add your own sweetness with fruit or honey. If you really prefer to stick with full-fat dairy, this is fine too.

Are products such as Weet-Bix and All-Bran cereal considered packaged food?

Yes. Even though they are wholegrain-wheat based, it is impor-tant to bear in mind that such packaged products will also contain other added ingredients such as salt and added sugar and there are many more suitable breakfast-based options such as oats, avocado on wholegrain toast, or fruit and yoghurt. Try to stay clear of all processed cereal products because it's just as easy to make something from scratch.

Can I eat any type of nuts and seeds?

Yes, you can enjoy a range of nuts and include a mix, such as walnuts and almonds. Choose dry-roasted or those in their natural form, without added oil or salt.

Are activated almonds better for me than normal almonds?

No! 'Activation' does not improve the digestibility and nutrition of the nut, despite all the clever marketing.

Can I drink soda water in place of water? Does soda water contain sugar?

You should focus your fluid intake on water and have soda water when dining out (it makes you feel like you are treating yourself to something other than alcohol). However, a suitable alternative is to make your own soda water at home and add some fresh lime – another one of nature's treats. Commercially bought soda water does not contain sugar but it does contain sodium, so don't have it as your primary source of fluid. Even mineral or sparkling water can contain sodium, depending on the brand, so be sure to check what you're buying if you're drinking it every day. And for those who drink tonic water, this also contains sugar, so if you must have it, stick to the 'diet' option. Remember, it's a treat too.

Do I have to cut out alcohol?

Only if you're pregnant or breastfeeding. If you want a drink when breastfeeding, pump and store the milk before having one. You can then feed your baby expressed milk from a bottle. Otherwise, the general rule is that no foods or drinks need to be cut from the IWL plan. If you enjoy it, you can include it. And you can have it in addition to your treat meal each week.

Studies tell us that alcohol leads to a small increase in your good high-density lipoprotein (HDL) cholesterol, but this only happens at low-level intake – no more than two standard drinks per day. You can also increase your HDL-cholesterol through regular physical activity. In practical terms, you should keep your intake to one average-size drink per day, because we tend to fill our glasses quite high (which equates close enough to two standard drinks). You should also include a minimum of two alcohol-free days per week. When consumed at levels above this recommended intake, alcohol can disrupt your sleep quality and may lead to a disinhibition of your appetite signals and subsequent poor food choices. It will also make it hard to lose weight during a weight-loss month, because alcohol is energy dense and it's the first fuel to be metabolised by the liver in the body, meaning that when you go and eat a meal afterwards it may end up getting stored as fat. Most people following the IWL plan say that they get away with including one glass of wine per night (approximately five nights per week) and still lose weight on the weight-loss months.

Is it bad to eat carbs at night?

No, you should eat carbs with every meal. Choose the wholegrain types to ensure every meal is balanced and help you feel fuller for longer. There is no research to suggest that carbs at night make you put on weight. That's just your friend proclaiming to be a so-called 'expert' on all things health. Stop listening!

I don't have the time to prepare lunch every day. Can I take the same thing every day?

Yes, you can. But, easier still, the IWL plan advocates for people to cook extra every night so that you always have leftovers for lunch the next day. If this doesn't work for you and you are convinced you will eat the whole damn lot even after it's packed away in the fridge, yes, you can make the same lunch each day. But it strongly suggests to me that you are not following the principles of the IWL plan, particularly the tunnel plan of big to small meals throughout the day. If you don't eat enough at the start of the day, you will always be hungry at the end of the day. And if you're bored and find yourself 'comfort' eating, get cracking on your to-do list.

Is a sandwich okay to take to work for lunch?

Yes, this is a great lunch option. If the sandwich incorporates a wholegrain carb, a protein source, a healthy fat source, and plenty of veg or salad, it gets the IWL tick of approval. Despite what some of your colleagues might think (and comment), sandwiches are healthy. Let them eat their keto meal or paleo plate of meat – you just need to worry about yourself and stick to the IWL plan. Good sandwich toppings include egg, lettuce, salmon, chicken, tomato, capsicum, spinach and so on – get creative!

Can I make my favourite dinners on more than one night per week?

Yes, of course. Routine and repetition are great if it's a healthy option, nutritionally balanced and you love it, as per the principles of the IWL plan. Research has shown that we make over 200 food choices a day, so make it a little easier on yourself and repeat the same meals. We certainly do in our household.

Is it a good idea to have a juice cleanse every so often to detox?

A juice cleanse or detox is not needed to cleanse your body of toxins. There is no such thing as a detox. This is nothing more than clever marketing. The body does this process on its own – just don't feed it a diet based on processed food all the time and include plenty of wholesome and nutritious foods as per the IWL plan. Leave the juicing for the Hollywood celebrities.

Should I only be eating 'clean' foods?

Clean eating means nothing; it has done nothing except contribute to the ever-growing diet industry and it's a very clever money maker. The reason it grabs people's attention is because it's catchy. Worryingly, it has morphed into a misleading phrase that has led people to think certain fruits and vegetables are bad; that carbohydrates are evil; that you should eat gluten-free; that coconut oil is a miracle food; and that you should obsess about every little ingredient. Don't get caught in the trap of listening to your friends; stay focused on what you are setting out to achieve with the IWL plan.

Should I take supplements? If so, which ones?

It is beyond the scope of this book to review all supplements that are currently available on the market; there are thousands of them, so if I haven't mentioned it you don't need to waste your money on it. This includes probiotics and specially marketed foods that are high in whatever they're marketed to be high in (you can get what they're flogging from food itself).

If you are eating all the foods suggested in this book you will *not* need supplements (except during pregnancy). This includes multivitamins. You will just end up excreting the vitamin supplements through your urine. For example, an excess of vitamin B2 (riboflavin) will be detected by a dark fluorescent urine colour. However, if you are a vegan or attempting to fall pregnant, there are certain supplements that you should take. Refer to the third principle of the IWL plan – *Full rainbow* – in which I outline the key nutrients of concern when following a vegan diet.

Before and during pregnancy you will need a folate supplement. You need 400 micrograms every day from when you are attempting to conceive until you're 12 weeks' pregnant to help with the healthy development of the spine and brain in the baby. Not everyone plans their pregnancy, so it's important in this instance to be taking a folate supplement from the time you know you are pregnant. Iron, calcium, iodine and vitamin D supplements may also be required during pregnancy, but only in consultation with your doctor.

You might consider some of the following supplements.

Iron

If you are planning a family or you do not get iron from animal sources (such as meat), an iron supplement is likely needed. Red meat is the richest source of bio-available iron and should be included in your food plan twice a week. Symptoms of low iron include tiredness and lack of energy. A deficiency can be detected through an iron-studies blood test by your doctor, which you should do before taking any supplements.

Calcium

If you avoid dairy or are not getting enough calcium-rich sources other than dairy (for example, tinned fish with bones, tofu and almonds) in your diet, you may need to include a calcium supplement. Calcium is important for bone health and preventing osteoporosis, also known as brittle bones. Dairy foods are the richest source of calcium and are of the highest bio-availability, meaning there is a higher absorption rate of calcium from the food. If you eat dairy or consume calcium-enriched plant sources of dairy (such as soy), you do not need this.

Vitamin D

In conjunction with calcium, vitamin D is also important for bone health and preventing osteoporosis. Natural sunlight is the richest source of vitamin D and we only require very small amounts each day. A five- to 10-minute walk outside each day will be enough to meet daily requirements. Vitamin D is also found in some food sources, such as eggs. However, for those who see little to no sunlight, a vitamin D supplement will most likely be needed. Please consult with your general practitioner before taking a supplement.

Omega-3

There are health benefits associated with omega-3 consumption specifically relating to a reduction in inflammatory markers in the body. However, research shows that the best way to get these anti-inflammatory benefits is to eat foods rich in omega-3, such as fish, or plant-based sources such as nuts and seeds. If you don't eat fish, you *may* benefit from a fish-oil supplement, but you need to be taking 3000 milligrams per day (usually three to six tablets per day depending on the strength you buy). Omega-3 fats are also important during pregnancy so, again, if you're not eating fish, a supplement is likely required. Make sure to store them in the fridge to prevent them oxidising.

Vitamin B12

If you are vegan or are deficient in intrinsic factor (an enzyme required to bind vitamin B12 in the stomach, with deficiency most common in those over 70) you will need a vitamin B12 supplement. Vitamin B12 levels can be detected by a blood test. If you fall into one of these categories (vegan or over 70 years of age) you should consult with your general practitioner for a subcutaneous injection or appropriate supplement.

Glucosamine

There is some clinical evidence to support the use of glucosamine for improving joint health. For those with a history of, for example, knee or hip pain, benefit may be gained from a daily supplement of glucosamine at an intake of 2000 milligrams per day.

Are superfoods any good?

The term 'superfood' has gained enormous traction and popularity because after all, it's something we all want – a food that promises to be super healthy so we can continue with our unhealthy lifestyle habits. All we need to do is add in some acai berries, chia seeds, kale, coconut oil or some almond milk. Acai berries, for example, are packed with antioxidants, vitamins and minerals, but so too are all berries, so it doesn't matter which ones you have. Kale also contains plenty of vitamins, minerals and antioxidants but you don't get any extra superpowers from eating kale than what you get from any other vegetable. All vegetables contain varying amounts of vitamins and minerals and they all give us superpowers. As for the plethora of other cleverly marketed superfoods, don't get caught up in the hype – you will get all the benefits they promise from the foods prescribed in the IWL plan and you will save a lot of money in the process.

How do I lose the weight off my tummy and hips?

This is referred to as 'spot reduction' and unfortunately there is no such thing, despite what you might see in those late-night TV ads promising to shrink your stomach. You can't lose weight in one specific spot. When you lose weight, it comes off the entire body. The tummy, hips and thighs are the stubbornest areas of all and often the last to see change. Your body will continue to change over time on the IWL plan but don't expect your tummy to disappear or your hips to shrink from doing lots of crunches or sit-ups.

Should I exercise in the morning or evening?

Exercise when it suits you. It doesn't matter when you do it, all that matters is you do it. Yes, I can hear many of you saying, 'I've heard it's best to exercise first thing in the morning before breakfast.' Well, you guessed it, this isn't true, and you're not going to burn more fat in the morning on an empty stomach.

Should I eat before or after exercise?

The principles of the IWL plan always apply – that is, big to small throughout the day and regular meals to avoid excessive hunger setting in. However, in saying this, it is not practical to have a large

meal before exercising – you are likely to feel ill and uncomfortable and you won't be able to train at the intensity you hoped. If
you prefer to exercise first thing in the morning, have something
very light before your activity (if you can tolerate it) and make sure
to eat as soon as you finish so that you stick to the principles of the
plan.

Will weights make me big?

No, weight or resistance training adds variety to your exercise
routine and will not result in you putting on weight or gaining
bulky muscle.

Apart from my body weight, what else should I be measuring?

You should have your height accurately measured so you can
calculate your BMI (your general practitioner can help with this).
The BMI is your weight over your height squared. There are lots
of online calculators that you can use after you accurately measure
your height and weight for the first time. One suitable example is
found at healthdirect.gov.au/bmi-calculator. BMI reference points
for males and females are:

Under 18.5	Underweight
18.5–24.9	Healthy weight range
25.0–29.9	Overweight
30.0 +	Obesity

However, there are many limitations of BMI; it doesn't account
for a person's muscle mass and hence why many athletes are incorrectly classified as overweight. The cut-off points were also derived

predominantly from data from North American and European populations and are not applicable to all ethnic groups. This issue has led to suggested redefined BMI cut-off points for people of Asian ethnicity (where a BMI of more than 23.0 is defined as overweight, and more than 27.5 as obese) and for those of Polynesian ethnicity, with a BMI cut-off point of more than 26.0 for overweight and more than 32.0 for obese.

It is a good tool to be used in conjunction with waist circumference. Your waist circumference should be measured by someone else to ensure an accurate measure. For consistency, the most accurate point of reference is the belly button. Ensure the measuring tape is square around the waist when the reading is taken. For women, work towards a goal waist measure of less than 80 centimetres and for men less than 94 centimetres. However, guidelines vary for different ethnicities. There are different guidelines for Asian, and South and Central American people, with a recommended cut-off of 80 cm for women and 90 cm for men.

You can also monitor your radial pulse and blood pressure. Your pulse can be taken on the radial artery, located on the lateral side of the wrist (just under the attachment of the thumb). The average normal pulse rate for males and females is 60–80 beats per minute. Athletes tend to have recordings between 40–60 beats per minute. If your pulse is above 80 beats per minute at rest, you should visit your GP for a health screen.

Your blood pressure can be taken by your general practitioner or with a digital machine that you can purchase from a pharmacy or department store. It is common to see high blood-pressure readings in those following an unhealthy lifestyle, and this will improve with weight loss. Ensure you are seated, have been resting for a few minutes, and that you are not talking when the measure is taken. A normal reading for males and females is 120/80. If it is above 140/90 you should visit your GP to have it checked.

If a weight-loss program is commercially available and large scale does this mean it can be trusted?

No, many of the weight-loss programs and products that are now available do not have any evidence to back up their claims. This includes commercial weight-loss programs that advertise heavily on TV. Many of these commercial providers just use testimonials and case studies on their websites to show how much weight people lose. This is not real research – this is anecdata, and anyone can post such claims about their product. With respect to the commercial programs that provide all your meals, just like every other diet, of course you will lose weight. You are eating meals that are calorie controlled, but as we all know it is not realistic to stay on this food forever. We get bored of it, it's expensive and repetitive and it's not a sustainable or educational approach to being healthy or to long-term weight loss. Plus, your body will end up fighting the weight loss.

PART 2

CREATIVE COOKING

This section of the book is intended to provide you with some examples of the types of meals you can include on the IWL plan. It is not intended to be a cookbook but instead give you some ideas of what you can cook, how easy it can be using just a few ingredients, and to show you what ingredients you should use as the foundations for all recipes. I'm not talking about laborious Michelin-star recipes that take hours to prepare. I'm talking about fun and easy recipes that anyone can cook, and, importantly, recipes the whole family can eat.

Cooking is a wonderful and fulfilling aspect of a healthy lifestyle as it encourages us to appreciate the food we eat. Not only will it ensure you are eating better, it will also save you money. It can be very easy if you stick to just a few ingredients and recipes that don't take all night to cook. Check the shopping list on page 79 to ensure you have all the core staples to hand. You shouldn't have to spend all afternoon at the supermarket looking for obscure ingredients and all evening in the kitchen cooking. No one has time to do that. Everyone can learn the basics of cooking – it just takes a little practice. It can be even easier if you have children, as they can be part of the cooking experience, which will teach them important life skills. Children as young as three years of age will benefit from this.

Much the same can be said when catering for the entire family. No one has the time to cook separate meals for different members of the family (and nor should they). It's fine to have all the family favourites, like spaghetti bolognaise; you just need to adapt them according to the principles of the IWL plan. For example, you would need to make sure your serve of spaghetti is served with salad or vegetables and that you tailor the portion size according to the meal of the day. Many of the recipes in this book can simply be mashed or thrown in the blender so your toddler can also enjoy them. That way you will only find yourself cooking one meal, instead of many!

With technology and social media platforms at our fingertips, there is no shortage of recipes that can be adapted to your IWL plan. Better still, you can sign up to my weekly recipe through the Interval Weight Loss website. The Interval Weight Loss online program also has new recipes each week.

A recipe is IWL friendly if it includes unprocessed or raw ingredients, plenty of vegetables (fresh or frozen) or salad, a lean protein source, a wholegrain carbohydrate and a healthy fat, such as extra virgin olive oil. There are times when convenience foods do play a role, such as pastry or stock, but it can be just as easy to cook simply with raw produce as it is to use pre-made ingredients. For example, making a basic pasta sauce from scratch is simple and far more nutritious than using a ready-made sauce from a jar. When it comes to seasoning with salt and pepper, most of us tend to overdo it, leading to an excess consumption of salt. To help wean yourself off this dependency, try making these recipes without the usual generous serving of salt you might use.

Even if you have never tried cooking, give it a go. Cooking is designed to be simple on the IWL plan.

My wife

A lot of the hard work that goes into testing these wonderful and easy recipes is done by my wife, Sally. We spend a lot of time in the kitchen making new IWL recipes to give you healthy and practical dishes that everyone can cook. Every week we devote time to making a new recipe and it's a lot of fun. Cooking doesn't need to be difficult and everyone can do it, but you must be willing to have a go.

Portion sizes

The serving size listed for each recipe is not gospel; rather, it is provided as a guide. You will notice that some recipes don't even give the number of serves. This is deliberate, as explained in depth in Part 1 of the book. Breakfast is the most important meal and you need to start monitoring your hunger signals so that you can adjust your food intake and portions as per the IWL plan. You will then need to taper off your food intake throughout the day so that lunch is the next biggest meal and dinner the smallest. Your evening meal should be served in a small rice-sized bowl or on a bread-and-butter plate, and preferably eaten with chopsticks or a teaspoon. It's also important to cook extra at each evening meal as this will go a long way towards ensuring success on your IWL plan. You should always have leftovers as these can be enjoyed for lunch the next day, saving you from having to look for healthy take-out options if you are not at home.

If you notice that your hunger is still higher before meals at the end of the day, you have some adjustments to make. Your body hunger signals don't change overnight, especially if you have been doing the same thing for decades (skipping breakfast and eating little throughout the day, only to have your biggest meal in the evening). This takes time to change, but if you do change your food structure and intake you will start to wake up hungrier in the morning, and you will feel better for it.

IWL community

Some of the recipes in this book are attributed to members of the IWL community. These are some of their favourite crafted IWL recipes that they wanted to share with others. Sharing nutritious simple-to-make food ideas is a great way of showing how easy it can be to succeed on this plan. Remember, if it includes a lean protein source, a wholegrain carb, a good source of fat, and some vegetables, it gets the IWL tick of approval.

Fresh vegetables and herbs

There's a lot to be said for growing your own vegetables and herbs, and you don't need a big garden to do so. Some of the best veggie gardens I have seen are grown on cleverly configured green walls in small apartments. Having your own veggie garden doesn't require much effort and just a little maintenance will ensure you have an ongoing supply of fresh produce at your fingertips. The only exception is if your place doesn't get any sun – then you will struggle to grow your own produce.

The core staples of any basic garden should include rosemary, basil, parsley, shallots, coriander and rainbow spinach or another leafy green such as kale, baby spinach or rocket. Mint is another handy one to grow as it is good for warding off bugs and flies. Be careful though as it behaves like a weed and can take over your entire veggie garden. These herbs are easy to grow and will often thrive with some sunlight, water and good nutrient-rich soil. Don't buy the cheap potting mix as it will only ensure failure; invest in a good-quality vegetable soil.

Picking your own fresh produce is extremely satisfying and, especially if you grow everything from seed, extremely cost-effective. Think about all those times when we buy expensive fresh herbs from the supermarket, only to use a small quantity and see the rest go to waste. Having your own veggie garden is also a great way to involve your children. Handing them the responsibility for picking the crops is a way for them to contribute to the family meal.

Visit your local nursery for advice about what you can grow in your home environment and which soil to use. Start small and expand your collection of herbs as you gain understanding about what grows best and at what time of the year. For those who develop a green thumb, the range of growing opportunity is endless. Tomatoes are a wonderful and easy form of produce to grow and you will notice they taste much sweeter than anything you buy from the supermarket.

QUICK AND EASY 'SAVE THE SITUATION' RECIPES

We all have times where we find ourselves caught short due to an unexpected event or a busy day at work. When this happens, it is much better to save the situation with one of these simple suggestions, rather than stopping for a burger and chips on the way home. Even if it means picking up a hot chicken. Yes I know, a hot chicken from your local takeaway is not the healthiest option, but it's a hell of a lot better than grabbing Maccas at the drive-through. Just stay clear of the chips. Grab some tabbouleh or other salad vegetables to go with it or use what you have in your fridge at home. A bag of greens will more than suffice. Toasted sandwiches are another great option and a wonderful way to save the situation while still sticking to the principles of the IWL plan.

Here are some of my other favourites.

NO-RECIPE PESTO PASTA

This is a perfect weeknight meal when time is at a premium and you are 'hangry'. These ingredients are entirely adaptable so just use what's in your fridge. We like it with something a bit salty, like olives, capers or anchovies, but everything else is negotiable.

1 packet wholegrain pasta, or whatever pasta you have on hand
fridge items (olives, capers, anchovies, sun-dried tomatoes, basil,
    kale, rocket, capsicum, zucchini, onion, garlic, tomato, cauliflower –
    whatever you like and have on hand)
1 jar of pesto (bought or homemade; see page 346)
sea salt and freshly ground black pepper

1. Cook the pasta according to the packet instructions.
2. Meanwhile, combine your fridge-raid ingredients in a large frying pan over medium heat. Add the pesto and stir to combine.
3. Drain the pasta, then toss through the ingredients in the pan. Season lightly to taste and enjoy!

QUINOA AND VEGETABLES

My wife and I often have a variation on this for lunch. It's cheap, nutritious and very filling. To speed things up, we roast a pile of vegetables on a Sunday or one evening after work, then portion them out during the week. You could also buy frozen vegetables, salad vegetables that don't need cooking (like a kaleslaw mix) or you could microwave the wholegrains to save on cooking time. Although not eco-friendly, a lot of wholegrains come in pre-cooked packets and you simply need to heat them up in the microwave.

Serves 2

1 cup uncooked quinoa, brown rice or similar

1 cup vegetables (roast sweet potato, cauliflower, pumpkin or zucchini; boiled or steamed broccoli, carrots, beans, corn, cherry tomatoes, avocado, etc.)

salad mix

½ cup protein (tinned chickpeas, chicken, tofu or similar – a pre-roasted chook will save you time or cook one on the weekend to use in lunches for the next few days)

2 tablespoons olive oil

condiment of your choice (pesto, hummus or another dip, hot sauce or similar)

optional extras (olives, capers, semi-dried tomatoes, cornichons)

1. Cook everything according to the packet instructions. If you are roasting veggies, spread them out on a baking tray with olive oil and roast in a preheated 180°C oven for 25 minutes or until tender and golden.
2. Mix everything together and divide up for lunches throughout the week.

KALESLAW AND SARDINES

This tasty combination takes all of 3 minutes to prepare. Just the thing when you have a late finish and can't be bothered to cook.

Serves 2

2 large handfuls of kaleslaw or similar
2 tins of sardines, drained
squeeze of sriracha sauce

Tip the kaleslaw into bowls or lunch containers, put the sardines on top and finish with a squeeze of sriracha.

BREAKFAST

B reakfast is the most important meal of the day and will be your largest on the IWL plan. You may not currently do this, but it's a great idea to start including vegetables because otherwise it can be quite challenging to meet the recommended five serves of vegetables or salad per day. It's not always practical to sit down to a big breakfast, and if you're working you may need to have something before leaving home and then another breakfast when you get to the office. Wholegrain toast, oats, fruit, yoghurt and eggs are all wonderful breakfast options that don't take a lot of time.

Making a large batch of muesli on the weekend is a great way to prepare for the week ahead. Line a baking tray with baking paper. Mix together 1 kg rolled oats, 1 cup unsalted nuts (dry-roasted or raw), 2 tablespoons seeds and 1 tablespoon ground cinnamon, spread out on the tray and bake for 15 minutes or until crisp and lightly golden. Store in a large container and use it for breakfast throughout the week. It goes well with fresh berries, honey and yoghurt.

My wife doesn't like most breakfast foods, so normally has leftovers or baked veggies for breakfast – also a great option.

Stephanie is a member of the IWL community. She has a real love for cooking, and these are some of her favourite breakfast recipes to satisfy her sweet tooth. She has learnt to retrain her brain by including plenty of nature's treats.

These breakfast suggestions are also very cost-effective as they use a lot of the same base ingredients, so you don't have to spend extra money buying one-off ingredients, only to use a small amount and waste the rest.

For these breakfast recipes, you can use whichever berries you prefer – strawberries, raspberries, blueberries, blackberries or mulberries, either fresh or frozen. And the riper the banana the better. You will often find the ones that are turning brown are sold cheaply for quick sale.

STEPHANIE'S BANANA BERRY OATS THREE DIFFERENT WAYS

Porridge
Serves 2

80 g rolled or steel-cut oats
2 bananas, lightly mashed
½ cup your choice of berries
1 medjool date, pitted and finely chopped
½ teaspoon vanilla bean paste
200 g natural or Greek yoghurt
100 g mixed nuts and seeds

1. Combine the oats, bananas, berries, date, vanilla and 1 cup (250 ml) water in a saucepan.
2. Bring to the boil over high heat, then reduce the heat and simmer, stirring regularly, for 3–5 minutes or until the porridge is thick and creamy.
3. Serve with yoghurt and a scattering of nuts and seeds.

Tip: You can keep one serve in the fridge (without the toppings) and gently reheat the next day. Just add a splash of water to the pan as it will have thickened on standing.

Overnight oats
Serves 2

⅔ cup (60 g) rolled or steel-cut oats
1 tablespoon chia seeds
2 teaspoons cashew or almond butter (or other nut butter)
½ cup (125 ml) skim milk
2 bananas, mashed
3 tablespoons berries (any variety but strawberries work particularly well)
2 teaspoons ground cinnamon
½ teaspoon vanilla bean paste
passionfruit pulp and an extra handful of berries, to serve (optional)

1. Place the oats, chia seeds, nut butter, milk, banana, berries, cinnamon, vanilla and ½ cup (125 ml) water in a bowl and mix together well.
2. Spoon into separate bowls or containers and refrigerate overnight.
3. When you're ready to eat, top with extra fruit, such as passionfruit and fresh berries, and serve.

Tips: Take it out of the fridge when you first wake up and allow it to come to room temperature. You can make this the same day if you have time to leave it for a minimum of 1 hour before eating.

You can also make a simple version of overnight oats with ½ cup (125 ml) milk or natural yoghurt, ⅔ cup (60 g) rolled or steel-cut oats, and a generous handful of frozen berries. Combine all the ingredients in an airtight container the night before and place in the fridge, then grab on your way to work the next day. Healthy, filling, cheap and delicious!

Oatmeal bakes

Makes 12

These have a dense texture, closer to a pudding or frittata than a muffin. They are delicious on their own but also go well with natural yoghurt.

4 bananas
4 eggs
80 g rolled or steel-cut oats
1 teaspoon vanilla bean paste
3 tablespoons berries (any variety but raspberries are great here)
olive oil spray
100 g natural yoghurt (optional)

1. Preheat the oven to 180°C.
2. Place the bananas, eggs, oats and vanilla in a bowl and mix until the banana is completely mashed and everything is well combined. Finally, fold in the berries.
3. Spray a standard muffin tray with olive oil, then spoon the batter evenly into the holes.
4. Bake for 25–30 minutes or until cooked through. Serve warm or cold with yoghurt, if desired. They keep well in the fridge for up to 3 days.

STEPHANIE'S 'ANY GRAIN YOU LIKE' PORRIDGE

You can make this with any kind of wholegrain – steel-cut or rolled oats, brown rice, wheat berries, spelt berries, farro, barley, freekeh. Each will give a slightly different flavour and texture, which is why this is one of Stephanie's favourite breakfast options.

Serves 1

40 g wholegrain (any variety)
½ cup (125 ml) skim milk
1 medjool date, pitted and finely chopped
½ teaspoon ground cinnamon
fresh or tinned fruit in natural juice, cut into bite-sized pieces, to serve
30 g unsalted nuts
100 g natural yoghurt

1. Cook the wholegrain according to the packet instructions. (Stephanie puts it on to cook as soon as she wakes up.)
2. Combine the cooked wholegrain, milk, date, cinnamon and ½ cup (125 ml) water in a small saucepan and simmer over low heat, stirring regularly, for 3-5 minutes or until you have a creamy porridge.
3. Top with your choice of fruit, nuts and yoghurt and enjoy warm.

Tip: Double or triple the quantities to make a large batch, so you can store and reheat later.

SOUPS AND SALADS

ROAST CAPSICUM AND TOMATO SOUP

As is often the case with soup, this recipe is a good way to use up any vegetables in your crisper drawer. It's also easy as anything. If you're like me, you often leave the odd ingredient out of a recipe to save a trip to the supermarket. Usually that's fine, but don't be tempted to skip the basil in this one – it really makes it!

Serves 6

2 red capsicums, seeds and membrane removed, quartered
4 large tomatoes, halved (look for the ones that are reduced to clear at
    your local greengrocer, specifically to use in soups)
olive oil, for cooking
generous drizzle of balsamic vinegar
2 garlic cloves, finely chopped (or 2 teaspoons jarred minced garlic)
2 red chillies, finely chopped (or 2 teaspoons jarred minced chilli)
1 brown onion, diced
2 cups (500 ml) salt-reduced vegetable or other stock
1 x 400 g tin tomatoes
2 potatoes (any variety), cut into small pieces
2 teaspoons tomato paste
1 cup (220 g) dried soup mix
large handful of basil leaves, roughly chopped
freshly ground black pepper

1. Preheat the oven to 180°C and line a baking tray with baking paper.
2. Place the capsicum and tomatoes on the prepared tray and drizzle with olive oil and balsamic vinegar. Roast for 30–40 minutes or until tender and lightly golden.
3. Shortly before the roast vegetables are ready, heat a drizzle of olive oil in a deep saucepan over medium heat. Add the garlic, chilli and onion and cook for 5 minutes.
4. Pour in the stock, add the tinned tomatoes, potato, tomato paste and soup mix and bring to the boil. Remove the roast vegetables from the oven and add to the soup pan. Simmer for 15 minutes or until everything is soft and well combined. Season with black pepper to taste. Scatter the basil over the top and enjoy.

Tip: If you like you can replace the soup mix with a 400 g tin of lentils, chickpeas or beans, drained and rinsed. This will reduce the cooking time if you are using the tinned variety.

SPICY (OR NOT!) CHICKEN NOODLE SOUP

This recipe is a delight – it's full of flavour, you can customise it to suit your palette and it's quick and easy to cook.

Serves 4

1 tablespoon olive oil
2 teaspoons finely chopped/grated ginger
4 garlic cloves, finely chopped (or 1 tablespoon jarred minced garlic)
500 g chicken mince
2 tablespoons chilli paste or 1 red chilli, finely chopped, or to taste
1 teaspoon sesame seeds

Broth
1 litre salt-reduced stock (any flavour)
2 heaped teaspoons white or yellow miso paste
⅓ cup (80 ml) soy sauce
2 carrots, cut into bite-sized pieces
1 brown onion, finely chopped
large handful of kale leaves, stems removed
250 g egg noodles

1. To make the broth, combine the stock, miso paste and half the soy sauce in a large saucepan over medium heat. Add the carrot and onion and bring to the boil, then reduce the heat and simmer for 10 minutes or until the carrot is tender. Stir in the kale and noodles.
2. Meanwhile, heat the olive oil in a frying pan over medium heat. Add the ginger and garlic and cook for 2 minutes. Add the chicken mince and cook, breaking up any lumps with the back of a wooden spoon. Stir in the chilli and cook for 6 minutes or until the chicken is lightly browned and cooked through.
3. Serve the mince into bowls and ladle the broth over the top. Finish with a light sprinkling of sesame seeds and serve.

FISH STOCK

This is a great recipe to make use of any leftovers after barbecuing a whole snapper (see page 298 for the barbecued snapper recipe), or any other whole fish. We store fish bones and skin in the freezer to make stock – it's environmentally friendly and good for the hip pocket!

If you are lucky enough to have a lot of leftovers from your barbecued fish you can make this into a soup by combining the strained stock with some chopped vegetables, such as potato, carrot, sweet potato, mushrooms and kale.

Makes 8 cups

1 kg fish leftovers (see Tip)
3 garlic cloves, chopped
1 white onion, chopped
6 sprigs flat-leaf parsley, chopped
freshly ground black pepper

1. Place all the ingredients and 2 litres water in a large deep saucepan over low heat. Simmer, covered, for as long as you can – it will be fine after an hour, but for a more intense flavour leave it on for longer – up to 4 hours.
2. Strain the stock, discarding the solids, and store it in the fridge for up to 4 days or the freezer for up to 3 months. Use it next time you're making anything that requires stock.

Tips: This is a guide only. If you buy your fish from the fishmonger, ask them to gut the fish and remove the gills as it makes for an easier and cleaner cooking process.

This recipe can also be adapted to use a chicken carcass.

ROAST VEGGIE SALAD

Like most IWL recipes, this can be customised to suit your taste and what's in your fridge. The veggies I've included here are the A team for this salad, but you could also roast tomatoes, carrots or zucchini. We like taking this camping or to people's houses – it travels well and doesn't require refrigeration for hours beforehand.

Serves 4 as a main or 6 as a side

1 large sweet potato, cut into bite-sized pieces
3 red capsicums, seeds and membrane removed, cut into thin strips
1 eggplant, cut into bite-sized pieces with sea salt sprinkled across
    the top
olive oil, for drizzling
1 x 400 g tin chickpeas, drained and rinsed
4 large handfuls baby spinach, rocket or basil leaves

1. Preheat the oven to 180°C and line a baking tray with baking paper.
2. Place the sweet potato, capsicum and eggplant on the prepared tray and drizzle with olive oil. Roast for 40 minutes or until tender and lightly golden. Remove and allow to cool slightly so they don't wilt the greens.
3. Place the chickpeas and greens in a salad bowl, add roast vegetables and gently toss to combine and serve.

Tip: You could also add capers, olives or fresh cherry tomatoes, or a grain like quinoa or couscous if you like.

GREEN SPRING-Y SALAD

This is really easy to make and delicious to eat, as well as being extremely cost-effective if you have a basil plant. You could also use fresh broad beans, edamame or peas.

Serves 8 as a side

1 cup (200 g) couscous
1 cup (200 g) frozen broad beans
1 cup basil leaves, roughly chopped
1 cup (100 g) walnuts, roughly chopped or broken by hand
100 g Danish feta, broken into bite-sized pieces

Dressing
1 cup basil leaves, roughly chopped
3 tablespoons white wine vinegar
1 tablespoon honey
2 garlic cloves, finely chopped
1 teaspoon dried chilli flakes
1 golden shallot, finely chopped
2 tablespoons olive oil

1. Cook the couscous and broad beans separately according to the packet instructions, then tip into a large salad bowl. (Make sure you pod the beans if necessary.) Add the basil, walnuts and feta.
2. To make the dressing, put all the ingredients in a food processor and blitz until combined.
3. Add the dressing to the salad immediately before serving. Enjoy!

SMOKED TROUT AND RISONI SALAD

Risoni is small rice-shaped pasta, also called orzo. It makes a wonderful accompaniment to the trout in this dish.

Serves 4

150 g risoni
1 tablespoon olive oil
200 g smoked trout
½ red onion, finely chopped
1 spring onion, finely chopped
2 tablespoons finely chopped rocket or watercress
2 tablespoons finely chopped flat-leaf parsley
about 12 green olives, pitted and chopped
finely grated zest of ½ lemon
2 teaspoons lemon juice
freshly ground black pepper

1. Cook the risoni according to the packet instructions (you want it al dente – not soft and mushy). Drain and toss through the olive oil. Set aside to cool.
2. Meanwhile, peel the skin back from the trout. Carefully lift pieces of the flesh away from the bone and break into small pieces, then place in a bowl. Turn the trout over and repeat on other side. Keep an eye out for any bones and discard them.
3. Add the onion, spring onion, rocket or watercress, parsley, olives and lemon zest to the risoni and toss to combine. Mix in the lemon juice and season with black pepper.
4. Add the trout and gently toss through, then serve.

CAULIFLOWER AND POMEGRANATE SALAD

This is a little bit fiddly, but it's a great one for entertaining. Have all the elements at room temperature and bring it all together just before you serve.

Serves 6

1 large head cauliflower
1 brown onion, diced
2 tablespoons olive oil
sea salt
½ cup (80 g) almonds
seeds of 1 pomegranate
juice of 1 lemon

1. Preheat the oven to 180°C and line a baking tray with baking paper.
2. Cut off one-third of the cauliflower and set aside for later. Place the remaining cauliflower (including the leaves) and onion on the prepared tray and drizzle with the olive oil. Season with salt and roast for 30 minutes or until tender.
3. Remove from the oven and cut the roast cauliflower into bite-sized pieces. Reserve the leaves for the salad – they look great and taste delicious.
4. Grate the reserved portion of cauliflower into a bowl. Add the baked cauliflower, almonds and pomegranate seeds. Drizzle the lemon juice over the salad and serve.

BROCCOLINI AND EDAMAME SALAD
WITH SESAME DRESSING

This speedy salad will go with just about anything – chicken, fish or a barbecue. It looks great and tastes amazing.

Serves 4

2 cups (500 g) frozen edamame
1 bunch broccolini, cut into bite-sized pieces
1 Lebanese or continental cucumber, cut into small pieces

Sesame dressing
⅓ cup (80 ml) soy sauce
1 tablespoon tahini
1 tablespoon sesame oil
1 tablespoon honey
sea salt, for cooking

1. Blanch the edamame and broccolini with a pinch of sea salt in a saucepan of boiling water for 5 minutes or until just tender. Drain.
2. Meanwhile, to make the dressing, place all the ingredients in a jar and shake to combine.
3. Combine the edamame, broccolini and cucumber in a bowl, add the dressing, season to taste and toss to coat.

MAIN MEALS

JAPANESE PRAWN PANCAKES

This recipe is fantastic with other seafood such as calamari, or similar. It's a quick and easy recipe that the kids will also enjoy cooking.

Serves 4

1½ cups (240 g) wholemeal flour
6 eggs
½ small green cabbage, shredded
500 g uncooked prawns, peeled and deveined, roughly chopped
3 tablespoons chopped spring onion
olive oil, for pan-frying

1. Put the flour in a bowl and gradually add 2 cups (500 ml) water, about ½ cup (125 ml) at a time, mixing well to avoid any lumps. Cover and chill in the fridge for 30 minutes.
2. Whisk in the eggs, one at a time, then stir in the cabbage, prawn and spring onion.
3. Heat a frying pan over medium heat and add a small splash of olive oil. Pour in one-quarter of the batter and cook for 3 minutes, then flip over and cook for a further 3 minutes, or until lightly golden and cooked through.
4. Remove to a plate and cover to keep warm while you cook the remaining pancakes.
5. Serve just as they are.

CHICKEN FILO PIE

Yes, you can still enjoy a pie on the IWL plan! Remember, you can enjoy all foods and recipes on the IWL plan – you just need to adapt them to the IWL way of life. In this instance, it is a healthier option to use filo pastry as opposed to puff pastry.

Serves 6

1 tablespoon olive oil
500 g chicken breast fillet, cut into bite-sized pieces
1 carrot, cut into bite-sized pieces
1 potato, cut into bite-sized pieces
½ cup (60 g) frozen peas
1 capsicum, seeds and membrane removed, cut into bite-sized pieces
3 spring onions, thinly sliced
250 g button mushrooms, thinly sliced
1.5 litres salt-reduced chicken stock
1 teaspoon finely chopped rosemary
1 teaspoon fresh thyme, or ½ teaspoon dried if you don't have any of
    the fresh variety
2 tablespoons wholemeal flour
2 teaspoons wholegrain mustard
4 sheets filo pastry
1 egg, lightly beaten

1. Preheat the oven to 180°C.
2. Heat 2 teaspoons olive oil in a large frying pan over medium heat. Add the chicken and cook, turning regularly, for 5 minutes or until just golden. Remove to a bowl.
3. Heat the remaining olive oil in the pan, add the carrot, potato, peas, capsicum, spring onion and mushroom and cook, stirring regularly, for 5 minutes.
4. Return the chicken to the pan and add the stock, rosemary and thyme. Sprinkle over the flour and stir to ensure there are no lumps.

Simmer for 10–15 minutes or until the vegetables are tender. Stir in the mustard halfway through the cooking time.

5. Line a large pie tin with three sheets of filo pastry. Scoop the chicken filling into the tin and fold the excess pastry in towards the middle. Place the remaining piece of filo on top and tuck it in to enclose the filling.

6. Lightly brush the top of the pie with beaten egg and bake for 15 minutes or until the pastry is crisp and lightly golden.

KOREAN HOT POT

If you can, it's good practice to cook rice from scratch. Try making large batches on the weekend and storing in the freezer until you need to use it. Alternatively, you can use the pre-cooked variety as this can be quite convenient on days where you are not prepared.

Serves 4

2 x 250 g packets pre-cooked black or brown rice
1 tablespoon olive oil
2 garlic cloves, finely chopped
1 carrot, cut into bite-sized pieces
500 g lean beef mince
1 red chilli, finely chopped
2 teaspoons sesame oil
1 tablespoon dark soy sauce (or light if that's what you have)
½ cup (100 g) kimchi
1 cup (80 g) bean sprouts
large handful of kale leaves, stems removed
olive oil spray
4 eggs
1 tablespoon sesame seeds
sriracha sauce or other chilli sauce, to serve (optional)

1. Prepare the rice according to the packet instructions.
2. Meanwhile, heat the olive oil in a large saucepan over medium heat. Add the garlic and carrot and cook for 1 minute, then add the beef mince, chilli, sesame oil and soy sauce. Cook, breaking up the mince with the back of a wooden spoon, for 5 minutes or until nicely browned. Add the kimchi, bean sprouts and kale, and stir for 1 minute to warm through, then remove the pan from the heat.
3. Spray a large frying pan with olive oil and heat over medium heat. Crack the eggs into the pan and cook, sunny side up, until the whites are set but the yolks are still runny.
4. Divide the rice among four bowls and spoon over the beef and vegetable mixture. Top each serve with an egg, sprinkle with sesame seeds and serve with chilli sauce, if desired.

OVEN-BAKED SALMON PARCELS WITH LEMON AND CAPERS

Fish can be a little challenging to cook but baking in the oven is a good way to retain its moisture and flavour. This is a delicious and easy dish to cook when you get home late as it only takes 10 minutes.

Serves 4

1 tablespoon olive oil
1 large head broccoli, cut into bite-sized pieces
250 g baby tomatoes
4 handfuls kaleslaw

Salmon parcels
4 x 150 g salmon fillets, with or without skin
4 slices lemon
1 tablespoon lemon juice
4 sprigs rosemary
1 tablespoon capers
sea salt and freshly ground black pepper

1. Preheat the oven to 180°C.
2. To make the parcels, tear off four square pieces of foil and place on the bench. Put a salmon fillet on each one and top with a slice of lemon, a drizzle of lemon juice, a sprig of rosemary and a few capers. Season to taste with salt and pepper, then wrap in the foil to firmly enclose the salmon. Place the parcels on a baking tray and bake for 10 minutes.
3. Meanwhile, heat the olive oil in a large frying pan over medium heat. Add the broccoli and stir-fry for 4 minutes, then add the tomatoes and kaleslaw and warm through.
4. Serve the salmon parcels with the vegetables.

BARBECUED WHOLE SNAPPER
WITH SWEET POTATO AND KALE CHIPS

The flavours of this dish make it a big hit with guests. Prepare everything before they arrive and put it on the barbecue 30–40 minutes before you're ready to eat.

Serves 4

1 x 1 kg whole snapper, scaled and gutted (see Tip)
4 garlic cloves, finely chopped
2 teaspoons grated ginger (or jarred minced ginger)
1 tablespoon chopped chilli (or jarred minced chilli)
olive oil
1 sweet potato, thinly sliced
4 large handfuls of kale leaves, stems removed
dried chilli flakes and garlic flakes, for seasoning
sea salt and freshly ground black pepper

1. Preheat your barbecue to medium.
2. Tear off a large piece of foil and place the snapper on top. Add the garlic, ginger and chilli to the mid-section (where the guts have been removed). Wrap the fish firmly in the foil.
3. Spray the barbecue plate with oil and add the fish parcel. Reduce the heat to low and cook for 30 minutes (keep an eye on the fish to make sure it doesn't dry out – it's cooked when the flesh is white and no longer clear). Keep the lid down and add the sweet potato chips after 10 minutes, remembering to turn them every so often.
4. Mix the kale leaves with a generous sprinkle of chilli and garlic flakes and season to taste with salt and pepper. Add to the barbecue when the fish is nearly cooked and let the leaves curl a little. Serve the fish with the sweet potato and kale chips.

Tip: Ask your fishmonger to gut the fish for you. It will save you a lot of time and effort, and won't cost any extra.

PRAWN, ASPARAGUS & SUGAR SNAP STIR-FRY

At IWL headquarters, we love prawns but sometimes struggle to be creative with them. Struggle no more with this quick, healthy and delicious take on a prawn stir-fry.

Serves 6

¾ cup (150 g) basmati rice
3 tablespoons olive oil
½ teaspoon sesame oil
2 garlic cloves, finely chopped
2 teaspoons grated ginger
6 spring onions, finely chopped
8 asparagus spears, sliced diagonally
150 g sugar snap peas, ends trimmed
1 kg uncooked prawns, peeled and deveined (see Tip)
1 lime, cut into 6 wedges

Sauce
3 tablespoons salt-reduced chicken stock
1 tablespoon soy sauce
1 teaspoon sugar (any type will do)

1. To make the sauce, combine all the ingredients in a small bowl. Set aside.
2. Cook the rice according to the packet instructions.
3. Meanwhile, heat a large wok or frying pan over medium heat. Add the oils, then the garlic, ginger and spring onion and stir-fry for 1 minute. Add the asparagus and sugar snaps and stir-fry for 1 minute.
4. Add the prawns and stir-fry for 1 minute or until they start to change colour. Pour in the sauce and toss to combine. As soon as the prawns are cooked, take the pan off the heat.
5. Spoon the rice into bowls and top with stir-fried prawns and vegetables. Serve with a lime wedge on the side.

Tips: A few pointers for preparing prawns:

Hold the prawn on its back and gently pull the head away from the body by snapping backwards.

Hold the prawn straight and gently pull the head away from the body; the black part (the digestive tract) will usually come out in one go. If it breaks off, gently pull it out with a toothpick.

Break off the legs until you reach the tail, then peel off the shell.

CRAB CAKES

You typically see crab cakes in the entree section of fancy seafood restaurants, making the idea of putting them together at home quite intimidating. However, they're easy to make and go well with the green spring-y salad on page 289, so you can turn them into a main dish.

Makes 8

1 egg, lightly beaten
1 teaspoon wholegrain mustard
½ teaspoon Worcestershire sauce
pinch of cayenne pepper
pinch of sea salt
pinch of freshly ground black pepper
300 g cooked crabmeat (see Tip)
½ cup (35 g) fresh breadcrumbs (see Tip), plus extra to coat
2 tablespoons finely chopped flat-leaf parsley
olive oil, for cooking
natural yoghurt, to serve

1. Combine the egg, mustard, Worcestershire sauce, cayenne pepper, salt and pepper in a large bowl. Mix in the crabmeat, breadcrumbs and parsley.
2. Spread extra breadcrumbs over a large dinner plate. Using wet hands, form the mixture into eight even balls and toss to coat in the breadcrumbs. Transfer to a clean plate, cover and refrigerate for 30 minutes.
3. Heat a splash of olive oil in a large frying pan over medium heat. Add the crab cakes, two to four at a time, and gently flatten with a spatula. Depending on the size of your pan you may need to cook them in two batches. Cook for 2 minutes each side or until heated through and nicely golden.
4. Serve warm with natural yoghurt.

Tips: Any frozen or fresh packaged crabmeat can be used here. You can also cook your own crabmeat if you wish, but this can be a laborious task.

Homemade breadcrumbs work perfectly in this recipe, as they do for any recipe that calls for breadcrumbs. Simply break up some stale bread and pulse in your food processor to form fine crumbs.

ROASTED EGGPLANT WITH PINE NUT SALSA

Oven-roasted vegetables are delicious, and this is another great one for the fortnightly menu. Just cut them up and let them bake away in the oven. Remember, not all recipes need to contain meat, and this is especially relevant during the weight loss months of the IWL plan.

Serves 4

4 large eggplants
2 eggs, lightly beaten
1 garlic clove, finely chopped (or 1½ teaspoons jarred minced garlic)
250 g baby tomatoes, quartered
1 cup wholegrain bread crumbs
finely grated zest and juice of 2 large lemons
⅓ cup (50 g) pine nuts, lightly toasted (see Tip)
small handful of basil leaves, chopped, plus extra leaves to serve
⅓ cup (80 ml) olive oil

1. Preheat the oven to 220°C and line a baking tray with baking paper.
2. Cut the eggplants in half lengthways and scoop out the flesh (they will look like little canoes). Place the eggplant shells on the prepared tray and put the flesh in a large bowl.
3. Add the egg, garlic, tomato and breadcrumbs to the eggplant flesh and crush the mixture together with a fork. Mix in the lemon zest, pine nuts, basil and 2 tablespoons olive oil.
4. Spoon the filling evenly into the eggplant shells and roast for 15–20 minutes or until they are lightly browned and the filling is cooked through.
5. Meanwhile, place the extra basil leaves in a bowl and dress with the lemon juice and remaining olive oil.
6. Remove the eggplants from the oven, top with the lemony basil and enjoy!

Tip: To toast the pine nuts, place them in a frying pan over medium heat for 2 minutes (or in the oven for a few minutes). Keep an eye on them as they can burn quickly. Remove them from the heat as soon as they are lightly golden.

STEAMED MUSSELS

This is such an easy meal to make and can be on the table in minutes. Make a trip to your local fish market or wholesaler and talk to them about your budget and the best time of year to buy them.

Serves 4

1 kg mussels, cleaned and debearded
4 tomatoes, chopped into bite-sized pieces
1 garlic clove, finely chopped
1 litre salt-reduced vegetable stock
wholemeal Lebanese bread, to serve

1. Place the mussels in a large saucepan, add the garlic and tomatoes, and pour over the vegetable stock.
2. Bring to a simmer and cook over medium heat for 6 minutes or until the mussels have opened (discard any that don't open). Serve with bread for dipping.

KIMCHI PRAWN STIR-FRY

This is a quick and easy weeknight meal, and quite adaptable to include whatever vegetables you have in the fridge.

Kimchi is a traditional fermented Korean dish. It is most commonly made with cabbage, salt and seasonings such as chilli, garlic and ginger. During the fermentation process, good bacteria convert carbohydrate into lactic acid, which preserves the vegetables and gives them their tangy taste. This 'gut-friendly' food has become increasingly popular in Western countries due to the recent interest in gut health, and it is readily available in larger supermarkets and Asian grocery stores. Fermented vegetables are a wonderful addition to your eating plan, but all vegetables and wholegrain carbohydrates will improve your gut health.

Serves 4

½ cup (100 g) kimchi
2 teaspoons grated ginger
1 teaspoon finely chopped garlic
2 tablespoons honey
2 tablespoons soy sauce
500 g uncooked prawns, peeled and deveined, tails intact
1 teaspoon olive oil
200 g egg noodles
1 cup vegetables chopped into bite-sized pieces (broccolini and green
    beans are great, but use what you have)
large handful of kale leaves, stems removed
2 spring onions, thinly sliced

1. Combine the kimchi, ginger, garlic, honey and soy sauce in a glass or ceramic bowl. Add the prawns and turn to coat, then leave to marinate for 10 minutes.
2. Heat the olive oil in a large wok or frying pan over medium heat. Add the chopped vegetables and, after a few minutes, add the

prawns (reserving the marinade for later) and cook for a further three minutes or until they curl and change colour.

3. Meanwhile, cook the noodles according to the packet instructions.

4. Add the marinade to the wok and mix to combine.

5. Divide the noodles among serving bowls, and spoon over the prawn and vegetable mixture. Top with spring onion and serve.

Tip: You could serve this with rice rather than noodles if preferred. Cook ½ cup (100 g) brown rice according to the packet instructions.

MISO FRIED RICE

This is a wonderful recipe that makes good use of any leftover vegetables you have in the fridge. Like most of our recipes, you can mix and match according to what you have. The miso adds a delicious umami flavour to the dish. The flavour and intensity can vary, so start with one teaspoon of miso paste and add more until it tastes right to you. You will find white, yellow, red and black miso on the shelves of major supermarkets. The darker the colour, the stronger the taste, so a red miso can overwhelm a mild dish like this.

Serves 4

1½ cups (300 g) brown rice
1 tablespoon white or yellow miso paste
1 tablespoon soy sauce or tamari (see Tip)
1 teaspoon sesame oil
3 tablespoons olive oil
3 eggs, lightly beaten
¼ brown onion
1 garlic clove, finely chopped (or 1½ teaspoons jarred minced garlic)
½ teaspoon grated ginger (or 1 teaspoon jarred minced ginger)
1 bunch broccolini or large handful of broccoli florets, cut into
    bite-sized pieces
1 red or green capsicum, seeds and membrane removed, cut into
    bite-sized pieces
3 large handfuls of green leafy vegetables (such as spinach or kale),
    roughly chopped
1 teaspoon oyster sauce

1. Cook the rice according to the packet instructions.
2. Meanwhile, place the miso, soy sauce or tamari and sesame oil in a small bowl and mix until smooth.
3. Heat 1 tablespoon olive oil in a large frying pan over medium heat. Pour in the egg and cook for 2 minutes or until the base is cooked, then flip over and cook briefly on the other side until the egg is just

set. Remove the omelette from the pan. (Don't worry if the egg sticks and your omelette doesn't slide out in one piece – it will still taste the same!)

4. Heat the remaining olive oil in the pan, add the garlic, onion and ginger and cook for 2 minutes. Add the broccolini and capsicum (and any other hard vegetables you may be including) and cook for a few minutes or until they start to soften.

5. Add the leafy greens, oyster sauce, rice and miso mixture to the pan and toss together until the greens begin to wilt, then remove from the heat.

6. Chop the omelette into thin strips and gently mix through the fried rice. Serve and enjoy!

Tip: Tamari and soy sauce are both made by fermenting wheat and soy and can be used interchangeably. Tamari contains less wheat and hails from Japan, whereas soy sauce comes from China.

ANDREW'S CHICKEN ENCHILADAS

This is one of my brother's favourite recipes! This tasty meal goes well with a side of guacamole or tomato salsa.

Serves 6

500 g chicken breast fillets, cut into bite-sized pieces
3 spring onions, thinly sliced
2 tablespoons teriyaki sauce
1 red capsicum, seeds and membrane removed, cut into thin strips
1 small red onion, finely chopped
100 g cheddar, grated
1 tablespoon olive oil
6 wholemeal wraps
2 tablespoons finely chopped coriander

Tomato salsa
small handful of coriander, roughly chopped
6 tomatoes, finely chopped
½ red onion, finely chopped
2 tablespoons lime juice
freshly ground black pepper

1. Place the chicken and spring onion in a bowl, add the teriyaki sauce and turn to coat well. Place in the fridge and marinate for at least 10 minutes.
2. Preheat the oven to 180°C and line two baking trays with baking paper.
3. To make the tomato salsa, combine all the ingredients in a bowl. Season with black pepper.
4. Place the capsicum, onion, 100 g salsa and 60 g cheese in a large bowl.
5. Heat the olive oil in a large frying pan over medium heat, add the chicken and cook for 3 minutes or until cooked through and no pink is evident. Scoop the chicken into the bowl with the capsicum mixture and toss to combine.

6. Divide the chicken mixture evenly among the wraps and roll up to enclose the filling. Place them on the prepared trays. Spread a tablespoon of tomato salsa across the top of each one and sprinkle over the remaining cheddar.

7. Bake for 10 minutes or until lightly browned and the cheese has melted. Top with remaining tomato salsa, sprinkle with some coriander and serve.

TAHINI–MISO VEGGIE BOWLS

Tahini – a Middle Eastern paste made of sesame seeds – gives this delicious dressing its creaminess, while the miso gives it a good kick of flavour. The dressing can also be used on chicken, steak, vegetables and other grains . . . the sky is the limit.

Serves 4

1 medium sweet potato or ½ small pumpkin, skin removed, cut into
　　bite-size pieces
1 cup (190 g) quinoa
3 tablespoons olive oil
250 g firm tofu, cut into bite-sized pieces
2 large handfuls of kale leaves, stems removed, roughly chopped
1 red capsicum, seeds and membrane removed, diced
sunflower seeds or similar, for sprinkling

Tahini dressing
½ cup (140 g) tahini
1 tablespoon white or yellow miso paste
1 teaspoon sriracha or other chilli sauce sauce, or to taste

1. Preheat the oven to 220°C and line a large baking tray with baking paper.
2. Spread out the sweet potato or pumpkin on the prepared tray with two tablespoons olive oil and roast for 30 minutes or until tender and golden.
3. Meanwhile, cook the quinoa according to the packet instructions.
4. To make the dressing, place all the ingredients and ½ cup (125 ml) water in a jar and shake to combine.
5. Heat the remaining olive oil in a large frying pan over medium heat. Add the tofu and cook for 3–4 minutes. Turn the pieces over, add three-quarters of the kale and cook for a further 3–4 minutes or until the tofu is golden and the kale has wilted.
6. Spread out the remaining kale on a baking tray and bake for 5–7 minutes or until crisp.

7. Divide the quinoa among four bowls and top with the capsicum, tofu, wilted kale and sweet potato or pumpkin. Drizzle over the dressing and finish with a sprinkling of sunflower seeds. Serve with the crisp kale chips on the side.

SALMON WITH SOBA NOODLES AND KALE

Many people don't like the skin of fish but it's a rich source of iodine. Iodine is essential for a healthy thyroid gland, which regulates our metabolism. Try keeping the skin on next time you cook as it also adds a different flavour to the dish, and texture, if a little crispy.

Serves 4

160 g dried soba noodles
2 tablespoons olive oil
1 garlic clove, finely chopped
2 carrots, chopped
2 spring onions, thinly sliced
2 tablespoons lemon juice
2 cups roughly chopped kale leaves
125 g cherry tomatoes, halved
3 tablespoons salt-reduced vegetable stock
4 x 120 g salmon fillets, with or without skin
2 teaspoons soy sauce
3 tablespoons roughly chopped coriander

1. Cook the noodles according to the packet instructions. Drain and rinse under water, then drain again.
2. Meanwhile, heat the olive oil in a large frying pan over medium heat. Add the garlic and cook for 30 seconds or until fragrant. Add the carrot and spring onion and cook, stirring regularly, for 3 minutes. Add the lemon juice, kale, tomatoes, stock, soy sauce and salmon and cook for a further 3–5 minutes or until the salmon is just cooked.
3. Divide the noodles among bowls and top with the salmon mixture, broken up into rough pieces. Sprinkle over the coriander and serve.

SALLY'S NASI GORENG

My wife Sally absolutely loves Asian food. If she could eat it every night, she probably would; so you would find her at the Indonesian restaurant and me at the Italian!

In our household, we use pre-cooked rice in emergencies – it's very convenient, but it's an eco-nightmare, and individual packets are going to cost you more. When we make recipes that require brown rice (like this one), we try to make double and freeze half for another time. But on days when we're not prepared, we use the emergency supply of individual pre-cooked packets.

As always, feel free to use other vegetables here. Good options include broccoli, broccolini, cabbage, baby spinach and even cucumber to serve.

Serves 6

3 cups (600 g) brown rice
2 tablespoons olive oil
1 garlic clove, finely chopped
1 white onion, finely chopped
3 carrots, cut into bite-sized pieces
½ head cauliflower, cut into bite-sized pieces
1 red or green capsicum, seeds and membrane removed, cut into
     bite-sized pieces
1 cup roughly chopped mushrooms
large handful of kale leaves, stems removed, roughly chopped
3 golden shallots, finely chopped
3 eggs
2 tablespoons soy sauce
3 tablespoons kecap manis (see Tip)
2 Roma tomatoes or similar, roughly chopped
3 teaspoons sambal oelek (see Tip)
1 cup (80 g) bean sprouts

1. Cook the rice according to the packet instructions.
2. Meanwhile, heat the olive oil in a large frying pan over medium heat, add the garlic and onion, and cook for 3 minutes or until lightly browned.
3. Going from the hardest to the softest, add the vegetables. So with the veggies listed above, you'd start with the carrot, then cauliflower, capsicum, mushroom and finally the leafy greens. The harder vegetables may take 8–10 minutes to cook and the softer vegetables just a couple of minutes.
4. Crack the eggs into the pan at the same time as you add the leafy greens and shallots, and mix into the vegetables. Cook for a further 2 minutes.
5. Mix together the soy sauce, kecap manis and sambal oelek in a small jug or bowl. Add to the pan, along with the tomato, and gently toss to combine.
6. Scoop into bowls and serve topped with bean sprouts.

Tip: Kecap manis is Indonesian sweet soy sauce. It's readily available at Asian grocers or at larger supermarkets. Sambal oelek is a Malaysian spice paste, also available in the Asian aisle at the supermarket. If you can't find it or don't want to buy it for just one recipe, feel free to use chopped fresh chilli or dried chilli flakes.

CAJUN CHICKEN BURGERS

I love burgers and this is my favourite chicken burger recipe. They are very quick and easy to make as well.

Serves 4

2 tablespoons olive oil
2 x 200 g chicken breast fillets, cut in half horizontally to make four
    pieces of equal thickness
4 wholegrain buns
1 avocado
250 g baby tomatoes, halved
3 pre-cooked baby beetroots (see Tip), sliced
2 large handfuls of rocket or baby spinach leaves
Cajun seasoning
1 tablespoon ground coriander
1 tablespoon ground cumin
1 tablespoon paprika, any variety
pinch of freshly ground black pepper
pinch of sea salt

1. To make the Cajun seasoning, mix together all the ingredients in a small bowl.
2. Rub 1 tablespoon of the olive oil all over the chicken pieces, then coat with the Cajun seasoning.
3. Heat the remaining olive oil in a large frying pan over medium heat, add the chicken and cook for 3 minutes on each side or until cooked through (the cooking time will vary depending on thickness of the breast).
4. Lightly toast the buns and spread a thick layer of avocado on each half.
5. Fill the buns with the chicken, tomatoes, beetroot and greens and serve.

Tip: You can buy pre-cooked, vacuum-sealed beetroot in the fresh produce section of the supermarket. If you're stuck, use 4 slices of tinned beetroot instead.

SAN CHOY BAU

Will you make a mess eating san choy bau? For sure. Will you also have fun? Guaranteed.

Serves 4

1 tablespoon olive oil
½ brown onion, finely chopped
2 garlic cloves, finely chopped
1 teaspoon finely grated ginger
1 small carrot, finely chopped
100 g tinned water chestnuts (optional)
750 g lean beef mince
1 iceberg lettuce, washed and outer leaves removed
crushed peanuts and bean sprouts, to serve

Sauce
3 tablespoons soy sauce
2 tablespoons oyster sauce
1 teaspoon sesame oil

1. Heat the olive oil in a large frying pan over medium heat, add the onion, garlic and ginger and leave to sizzle for 2 minutes. Add the carrot and water chestnuts (if using) and cook for a further 3–5 minutes. They should still be a little crunchy.
2. Meanwhile, to make the sauce, mix together all the ingredients in a small jug or bowl.
3. Add the beef to the pan and cook for 3–5 minutes or until nicely browned, breaking up any lumps with the back of a wooden spoon. Add the sauce and stir it through.
4. Pull leaves off the iceberg lettuce and fill each one with a spoonful of the meat mixture. Top with crushed peanuts and bean sprouts and enjoy.

FISH TACOS

This recipe has a few different elements, so it takes longer than most IWL recipes to prepare, but it's well worth it! The guacamole and pico de gallo can both be made ahead of time and stored in the fridge until you're ready to eat.

Serves 4

2 green or red capsicums, seeds and membrane removed, roughly
    chopped
1 tablespoon olive oil
500 g white fish fillets (such as ling), skin and bones removed
8 wholegrain tortillas

Pico de gallo
250 g cherry tomatoes, roughly chopped
small handful of coriander, chopped
½ red onion, diced
juice of 2 limes

Guacamole
2 avocados
sea salt, chilli or lime juice (optional – you can also just mash the
    avocado)

1. Preheat the oven to 180°C.
2. To make the pico de gallo, combine all the ingredients in a bowl.
3. To make the guacamole, mash the avocados in a bowl and add any
   other ingredients you like in your guac.
4. Heat a large frying pan over high heat, add the capsicum and cook
   until the skins begin to blister. Remove from the pan and peel off
   the skins, however its fine to leave them on if you prefer.
5. Heat the olive oil in the same pan, add the fish and cook for
   3 minutes each side or until just cooked through. It doesn't matter
   if it sticks a little bit and breaks as you will pull it apart to serve
   anyway.

6. Meanwhile, wrap the tortillas in foil and warm in the oven for
   5 minutes.

7. Put the pico de gallo, guacamole, capsicum, fish and tortillas on
   the table and let everyone make their own tacos. Best enjoyed with
   sangria!

SQUID INK PASTA WITH CALAMARI

Fresh squid ink pasta is a popular dish on the shores of Sicily, but dried squid ink pasta goes perfectly well with this dish and can be found at your local grocery store.

This spooky pasta would be a great idea for a Halloween gathering and is an absolutely stunning dish to look at, making it the perfect snap for Instagram. Make sure to include a photo of your squid ink pasta on the Facebook group or tag me on Instagram – @intervalweightloss – you'll go in the running for our weekly IWL prize. It doesn't just have to be this recipe; it can be any of them.

Serves 6

400 g squid ink spaghetti (spaghetti al nero di seppia)
½ cup (125 ml) olive oil
2 garlic cloves, finely chopped
1 tablespoon dried chilli flakes
1 tablespoon capers
1 x 400 g tin diced or chopped tomatoes
¾ cup (185 ml) salt-reduced chicken or vegetable stock
4 calamari tubes, cut into bite-sized rings
freshly ground black pepper
coriander or flat-leaf parsley leaves, to garnish

1. Cook the spaghetti according to the packet instructions.
2. Meanwhile, heat 3 tablespoons olive oil in a large frying pan over medium heat. Add the garlic and chilli and cook, stirring, until the garlic is lightly golden. Add the tomatoes and stock and simmer for 5 minutes.
3. Add the calamari rings and cook for a couple of minutes. They will curl when they are cooked.
4. Drain the pasta and rinse under hot running water. Tip the pasta into the frying pan and toss to combine with the capers and other ingredients.
5. Season with pepper, garnish with your choice of fresh herbs and serve.

Tip: This dish works very well using prawns as well.

GINGER AND MISO MARINATED
CHICKEN WITH CHARRED BROCCOLINI

Miso is a delicious addition to this recipe. Not only does it give the chicken a delicious seasoning, it also helps to create a smoky and charred texture when the chicken hits the grill. The wonderful creamy dressing completes the dish.

Serves 6

2 tablespoons white or yellow miso paste
3 garlic cloves, finely chopped
2 tablespoons finely grated ginger (or jarred minced ginger)
2 teaspoons sesame seeds
2 tablespoons sesame oil
2 chicken breast fillets (225g each)
1 bunch broccolini
large handful of kale leaves, stems removed

Tahini miso dressing
1 tablespoon white or yellow miso paste
1 tablespoon tahini

1. Combine the miso, garlic, ginger, sesame seeds and 1 tablespoon sesame oil in a glass or ceramic bowl. Add the chicken and massage the marinade into the meat. Cover and marinate in the fridge for at least 20 minutes – ideally up to 2 hours if time permits.
2. To make the tahini dressing, place the miso, tahini and 2 tablespoons water in a small bowl and mix together well. Set aside.
3. Preheat a stovetop cast-iron plate over medium heat or barbecue to medium. Add the remaining sesame oil, then the chicken and cook for 5 minutes. Turn the chicken over, add the broccolini and cook for another 5 minutes or until the broccolini is tender and lightly charred and the chicken is cooked through. The cooking time will vary, depending on the thickness of the breasts so they may need a little longer, though take care not to overcook them or

they will be dry. Make a small incision in the thickest part to make sure there is no pink evident.

4. Add the kale for the last couple of minutes of cooking time.

5. Remove the chicken and allow to rest for 2 minutes, before cutting it into thick slices. Drizzle with the dressing and serve with the broccolini and kale.

GRILLED SARDINES

Sardines are cheap, healthy and delicious, although they are not for
the faint hearted – these are a fishy fish! You can buy them gutted from
the fishmonger. To eat, chop the heads off the cooked sardines and
eat as is or use a fork to pull the flesh from the fish's spine. Serve with
some pan-fried vegetables of your liking.

Serves 2

8 sardines
sea salt
1 tablespoon olive oil

1. About 30 minutes before you are ready to eat, generously salt the
   sardines (I'd say six good grindings of your salt mill).
2. Heat a frying pan over high heat (or preheat your barbecue to high).
   After a couple of minutes, reduce the heat to medium and add the
   olive oil. Cook the sardines for 3–4 minutes each side.

BARBECUED KING PRAWNS

This is a quick, easy and healthy dinner. It may not suit everyone's budget but we have it every so often as a little treat. Serve with some pan-fried vegetables of your liking.

Serves 6

3 tablespoons soy sauce
1 tablespoon sesame oil
dried chilli flakes, for sprinkling
1 teaspoon honey
1 teaspoon finely chopped garlic
1 kg uncooked king prawns, peeled and deveined, tails intact

1. Mix together the soy sauce, sesame oil, honey, garlic and chilli flakes, to taste, in a glass or ceramic bowl. Add the prawns and turn to coat, then leave to marinate for 5–10 minutes.
2. Preheat your barbecue to medium. Cook the prawns for 1–2 minutes each side or until just cooked and serve immediately.

PUMPKIN AND QUINOA BURGERS

These can take a little while to prepare so are best saved for a day when you have some time up your sleeve. Alternatively, the pumpkin and quinoa can be cooked in advance.

Serves 4

4 wholegrain buns
½ avocado
2 handfuls of lettuce leaves (I love lamb's lettuce here but any variety is fine)
1 tomato, thinly sliced

Patties
500 g pumpkin, peeled and cut into bite-sized pieces
olive oil spray
3 tablespoons quinoa
¾ cup (75 g) walnuts
1 garlic clove, finely chopped
200 g tinned chickpeas, drained and rinsed
finely grated zest of 1 lemon
2 teaspoons ground cumin
freshly ground black pepper, for seasoning

1. To make the patties, preheat the oven to 180°C and line a baking tray with baking paper.
2. Spread out the pumpkin on the prepared tray and lightly spray with olive oil. Bake for 20 minutes or until tender when tested with a fork.
3. Meanwhile, cook the quinoa according to the packet instructions.
4. Place the pumpkin, quinoa and remaining patty ingredients in a food processor and blitz until combined. Season with black pepper. Form into four palm-sized patties, then cover and chill in the fridge for 10–20 minutes or until you are ready to cook them.
5. Spray a large frying pan with olive oil and heat over medium heat (or preheat your barbecue to medium). Cook the patties for 3 minutes each side or until golden and cooked through.
6. Split the buns in half and spread with the avocado. Add the patties, lettuce and tomato and serve.

CALAMARI WITH POTATO SALAD

Cooking with calamari is an inexpensive way to enjoy seafood, and this dish just melts in your mouth. It's always worth speaking to your local fishmonger about your best options – you will find them incredibly helpful and they will clean and gut the seafood for you too.

Serves 6

5 large potatoes (any variety), with or without skin
700 g calamari tubes, cut into thick rings
1 tablespoon olive oil
125 g baby tomatoes, halved
large handful of rocket
dressing
125 g baby tomatoes, halved
3 tablespoons olive oil
1 tablespoon capers
1 tablespoon wholegrain mustard
1 tablespoon red wine vinegar
1 garlic clove, finely chopped (or 1 teaspoon jarred minced garlic)
2 large handfuls of herbs and salad leaves (I like a mixture of flat-leaf
    parsley, rocket and basil but use what you have)

1. Boil the potatoes in a large saucepan of water for 20 minutes or until tender (they will begin to split).
2. Meanwhile, to make the dressing, place all the ingredients in a food processer and blitz to combine.
3. Place the calamari in a bowl, add half the dressing and toss to coat. Chill in the fridge until the potatoes are ready.
4. Drain the potatoes and cool slightly, then cut lengthways into 2 cm thick slices. Add the remaining dressing and mix until well coated.
5. Heat the olive oil in a large saucepan over medium heat. Add the calamari and its dressing and cook for 3 minutes or until just cooked through.
6. Divide the tomato, rocket and potato salad among plates, top with the calamari and serve.

SEAFOOD LINGUINE

This beautiful dish comes together really quickly. We use seafood marinara from our local fishmonger, but supermarkets also sell it if you don't want to make two stops. Of course, you can use whatever seafood you like – prawns, calamari or fish fillets all work a treat.

Serves 4

500 g linguine or pasta of your choice
1 tablespoon olive oil
5 garlic cloves, finely chopped (or use 1 heaped tablespoon jarred
    minced garlic)
1 red chilli, finely chopped, or pinch of dried chilli flakes
1 brown onion, diced
1 x 400 g tin chopped tomatoes
800 g seafood marinara, or similar
large handful of rocket, baby spinach or basil leaves

1. Cook the pasta according to the packet instructions. Drain.
2. Meanwhile, heat the olive oil in a large heavy-based saucepan over medium heat. Add the garlic, chilli and onion and cook, stirring, for 5 minutes or until softened and fragrant. Add the tomatoes and seafood and cook, stirring constantly, for 5–7 minutes or until the seafood is cooked. Stir in the greens.
3. Add the pasta to the seafood mixture and gently toss to combine. Serve hot.

ZA'ATAR LAMB PITA POCKETS

Za'atar is a popular Middle Eastern spice blend and is a wonderful accompaniment to meat, particularly lamb. It's easy to make your own, and we often do when friends come over – it's delicious served with extra virgin olive oil and pita bread.

Serves 4

600 g butterflied lamb leg, marinated if you prefer (see Tip)
1 tablespoon olive oil
100 g hummus (See Tip)
100 g beetroot dip (See Tip)
4 wholemeal pita breads
small handful of flat-leaf parsley or coriander leaves

Za'atar
1 tablespoon sesame seeds
3 teaspoons ground cumin
1 teaspoon dried oregano
1 teaspoon ground paprika, any type

1. Preheat your barbecue to medium or a stovetop cast-iron plate over medium heat.
2. To make the za'atar, combine the ingredients in a bowl.
3. Rub the za'atar all over the lamb.
4. Add the olive oil and lamb to the hot plate and cook for 3 minutes each side, turning once. Remove and rest for 5 minutes, then cut the lamb into thin strips.
5. Spread the hummus and beetroot dip into the pita pockets, add the lamb strips and fresh herbs and enjoy.

Tips: You can opt to buy lamb already marinated from your local butcher. Alternatively, you will also find pre-marinated vacuum-sealed packets of lamb at your supermarket.

There are good recipes for hummus and beetroot dip available on the IWL website. Otherwise, opt for commercial varieties of either dip.

SATAY SAUCE

This delicious peanut sauce is a good alternative to using the not-so-healthy trendy coconut products and is definitely healthier than store-bought sauce. It freezes well, and is particularly good with chicken and prawns, in a stir-fry or on noodles.

We usually have it with chicken skewers. Simply chop some chicken thigh or breast fillets into large bite-sized pieces and thread onto skewers. Grill them on the barbecue or cook them in a chargrill pan, and serve on a bed of thinly sliced cucumber and radish. A scattering of coarsely chopped coriander and mint leaves rounds out the freshness.

Serves 4

1 tablespoon canola oil
3 golden shallots, finely chopped
2 garlic cloves, finely chopped (or 2 teaspoons jarred minced garlic)
2 teaspoons grated ginger (or jarred minced ginger)
½ teaspoon ground turmeric
1 teaspoon chilli paste (or sliced fresh chilli or dried chilli flakes,
    to taste)
3 tablespoons lemon or lime juice
2 tablespoons soy sauce
1 tablespoon honey
3 tablespoons natural peanut butter
2 tablespoons milk

1. Heat the canola oil in a large frying pan over medium heat. Add the shallot, garlic, ginger, turmeric and chilli and cook for 5 minutes, stirring frequently.
2. Add the lemon or lime juice, soy sauce, honey, peanut butter and 3 tablespoons water. Bring to the boil, then remove from the heat and allow to cool for 2–3 minutes. Stir in the milk until creamy. Enjoy!

LEBANESE COUSCOUS WITH BREADCRUMBS, SUN-DRIED TOMATOES, ANCHOVIES AND CAPERS

This is my favourite recipe in this book! A big call I know, but it's simply delicious. The key ingredient is definitely the breadcrumbs, and while we use Lebanese couscous here, the dish goes extremely well with different varieties of couscous as well, such as whole-wheat pearl couscous. It's not as obscure as you might think – you will find it in all the big supermarket chains.

Serves 4

1 cup (140 g) Moghrabieh (Lebanese couscous)
1 tablespoon olive oil
3 tablespoons fresh breadcrumbs
1 cup basil leaves, roughly chopped
1 cup flat-leaf parsley, roughly chopped
3 tablespoons lemon juice
½ cup (60 g) pitted green olives, halved
2 tablespoons capers
30 g sun-dried tomato strips, without oil
10 small anchovy fillets, roughly chopped

1. Cook the couscous according to the packet instructions. Drain.
2. Meanwhile, heat the olive oil in a large frying pan over medium heat, add the breadcrumbs and cook, stirring regularly, for 1–2 minutes or until nicely golden.
3. Mix together the basil, parsley, lemon juice, olives, capers, sun-dried tomatoes and anchovies in a large bowl.
4. Add the couscous and basil mixture to the breadcrumbs. Reduce the heat to low and cook, stirring regularly, for 3–5 minutes or until well combined and heated through. Serve and enjoy!

MUSSEL AND TOMATO RISOTTO

You know what's better than slaving over a stove, constantly stirring? Throwing a pot of rice in the oven.

Serves 4

350 g baby tomatoes, any variety
1 brown onion, finely chopped
2 garlic cloves, crushed
1 tablespoon olive oil
sea salt and freshly ground black pepper
1½ cups (300 g) arborio rice
3 cups (750 ml) salt-reduced fish or vegetable stock
1 kg mussels, cleaned and debearded
large handful of baby spinach or kale leaves, stems removed
lemon wedges, to serve

1. Preheat the oven to 190°C.
2. Place the tomatoes, onion and garlic in a deep baking dish, drizzle with the olive oil and season with salt and pepper. Bake for 10 minutes.
3. Remove and stir in the rice and stock. Return to the oven and bake for another 30 minutes, stirring every 10 minutes.
4. Remove the dish and arrange mussels on the rice. Add the leafy greens and cover with foil or a lid and return to the oven for a further 15 minutes. Remove and discard any mussels that have not opened by the end of the cooking time.
5. Taste and season if needed, then serve with lemon wedges.

CHICKPEA PASTA

This is a great weeknight dinner when there's nothing in the fridge and everyone is starving. Almost all the ingredients are pantry staples!

Serves 4

2 tablespoons olive oil
3 garlic cloves, finely chopped
3 tablespoons tomato paste
sea salt
200 g tinned chickpeas, drained and rinsed
400 g small pasta
½ cup (125 ml) salt-reduced stock (any type) or water
1 small red chilli, finely chopped, or a generous shake of dried chilli
    flakes
1 sprig rosemary, leaves stripped, or generous shake of dried rosemary

1. Heat 1 tablespoon olive oil in a deep frying pan or large saucepan over medium heat, add the garlic and cook until lightly golden. Add the tomato paste and salt to taste, then cook, stirring, for 5 minutes. Add the chickpeas and cook for a further 5 minutes.
2. Add the pasta and pour in the stock or water. Simmer for 6–8 minutes or until the pasta is al dente. It's ready to eat now if you want more of a broth, otherwise continue cooking until thickened to a sauce consistency.
3. Stir in the chilli and rosemary, drizzle with the remaining olive oil and serve.

SALMON RISOTTO

This is a delicious and healthy way to eat salmon. It's fancy enough to serve dinner guests, and, aside from the greens, you'll find everything you need in your pantry or freezer.

Serves 4

2 tablespoons olive oil
1 brown onion, diced
2 garlic cloves, minced
250 g (1¼ cups) arborio rice
1 litre salt-reduced vegetable or fish stock
1 bunch broccolini, cut into bite-sized pieces
2 large handfuls of baby spinach, rocket or kale leaves, stems removed
2 x 120 g salmon fillets, with or without skin
juice of 1 lemon

1. Heat 1 tablespoon olive oil in a deep frying pan over medium heat, add the onion and garlic and cook, stirring, for 3–4 minutes or until fragrant. Add the rice and stir until the rice is coated with the oil and is almost transparent.
2. Pour in the stock. (When making traditional risotto you heat it first and add it in small batches while stirring constantly, but I like to live dangerously.) Cook, stirring occasionally, for 10 minutes or until all the stock has been absorbed. Add the greens and let them soften, then remove the pan from the heat.
3. Push the rice mixture to the side of the pan. Add the remaining olive oil and the salmon fillets and pan-fry for 5 minutes or until cooked to your liking.
4. Divide the risotto and salmon among four plates, finish with a squeeze of lemon juice and serve.

MEATBALLS

This family favourite is so easy to put together and can be on the table in half an hour. Serve with your choice of pan-fried vegetables.

Serves 4

500 g lean beef mince
1 sprig rosemary, leaves stripped
3 garlic cloves, finely chopped
1 egg, lightly beaten
1 teaspoon olive oil
1 x 400 g tin tomatoes
freshly ground black pepper, for seasoning

1. Place the mince, rosemary, garlic and egg in a bowl, season with black pepper and mix together well. With wet hands, form the mixture into golf ball-sized shapes.
2. Heat the olive oil in a medium frying pan over medium heat, add the meatballs and tomatoes and cook for 20 minutes or until the meatballs are cooked through. Garnish with a fresh herb or grind of freshly ground black pepper.

BAKED BROCCOLINI AND CANNELLINI BEANS

This is definitely, in my opinion, the best thing you can do with beans! Satisfying, very affordable and aside from the broccolini, everything comes from the cupboard!

Serves 4

3 garlic cloves, finely chopped
3 tablespoons extra virgin olive oil, plus extra for pan-frying
10 small anchovy fillets, finely chopped (optional)
1 teaspoon dried chilli flakes
1 x 400 g tin cannellini beans, drained and rinsed
2 bunches broccolini, cut into large bite-sized pieces
½ lemon, sliced
freshly ground black pepper
1 tablespoon grated parmesan
4 eggs
juice of 1 lemon

1. Preheat the oven to 180°C and line a large baking tray with baking paper.
2. Combine the garlic, olive oil, anchovies and chilli flakes in a large bowl. Add the cannellini beans and broccolini and gently toss to coat.
3. Spread the mixture evenly over the prepared baking tray, top with the lemon slices and season with black pepper. Bake for 15 minutes. Sprinkle over the parmesan and bake for another few minutes until the cheese has melted.
4. Meanwhile, heat a drizzle of extra olive oil in a frying pan over medium heat. Crack the eggs into the pan and cook until the whites are set but the yolks are still runny.
5. Remove the baking tray from the oven and drizzle lemon juice over the bean mixture. Spoon into four bowls and finish each serve with an egg on the top. Enjoy!

PESTO CHICKEN WITH PASTA

This is a very affordable meal that can easily be doubled or tripled for a larger group. Serve with a big green salad.

Serves 4

4 x 120 g chicken breast fillets
sea salt and freshly ground black pepper
3 tablespoon olive oil
2 tablespoons basil pesto (either bought or homemade; see page 346)
500 g pasta (any shape you like)
1 cup basil leaves, roughly chopped

1. Preheat the oven to 200°C.
2. Season the chicken with salt and pepper. Heat 1 tablespoon olive oil in a large ovenproof frying pan over medium heat, add the chicken breasts and cook for about 5 minutes each side or until nicely golden.
3. Slather the chicken breasts with half the pesto, then place in the oven and bake for a further 10 minutes or until cooked through.
4. Meanwhile, cook the pasta according to the packet instructions. Drain, reserving 3 tablespoons of the cooking water, and return to the pan. Add the basil, reserved water, remaining pesto and remaining olive oil and toss until a sauce forms and the pasta is well coated.
5. Divide the chicken breasts and pasta among plates and serve with a green salad.

Tip: For those who don't have an ovenproof frying pan, transfer the chicken into a large baking dish after cooking them initially in the fry pan for 5 minutes each side.

Robyn is a member of the IWL community and has always had a passion for cooking. On the IWL plan she learnt how to amend her favourite recipes by swapping various ingredients for healthier alternatives. These tweaks have enabled her to achieve her weight-loss goal and maintain it. We are delighted to share some of her favourite IWL recipes with you.

ROBYN'S HEALTHY MOUSSAKA STACK WITH LEMON AND YOGHURT DRESSING

Serves 2

1 large eggplant, sliced lengthways into 6 pieces
1 red capsicum, seeds and membrane removed, quartered
1 zucchini, sliced lengthways into 6 pieces
1 brown onion, finely chopped
1 large handful baby rocket

Meat sauce
1 small brown onion, finely chopped
1 garlic clove, crushed
½ stick celery, finely chopped
1 cup (250 ml) salt-reduced beef stock
170 g lean beef mince
2 tomatoes, roughly chopped
¼ teaspoon ground cinnamon
¼ teaspoon ground nutmeg
2 tablespoons roughly chopped flat-leaf parsley
2 tablespoons roughly chopped basil

Lemon and yoghurt dressing
3 tablespoons natural yoghurt
1 tablespoon finely grated lemon zest
1 tablespoon lemon juice

1. To make the meat sauce, heat a large frying pan over medium heat, add the onion, garlic, celery and half the stock and cook for a few minutes or until the onion has softened. Add the beef mince, tomatoes, cinnamon and nutmeg and cook, stirring and breaking up any lumps with the back of a wooden spoon, until nicely browned. Pour in the remaining stock and bring to the boil. Reduce the heat and simmer for 5 minutes or until the liquid has been absorbed. Remove the pan from the heat and stir in the fresh herbs.

2. Meanwhile heat another large frying pan or chargrill pan over medium heat and cook the eggplant, capsicum, zucchini and onion until browned and tender. Depending on the size of your pan you made need to do this in batches. (Alternatively, cook the veggies on the barbecue if you have it fired up.)

3. To make the lemon and yoghurt dressing, combine all the ingredients in a small bowl or jug.

4. Stack the eggplant, capsicum, zucchini, onion, rocket and meat sauce on serving plates. Drizzle with the dressing and serve.

Tip: When cooking this recipe, make double the quantity of meat sauce and freeze half to use in Robyn's beef taco recipe (see page 339). Simply thaw, reheat and add the kidney beans.

ROBYN'S BEEF TACOS WITH SALAD

Makes 10

1 quantity of Robyn's meat sauce (see the moussaka recipe on
    page 337)
3 tablespoons drained and rinsed tinned red kidney beans
10 jumbo taco shells

Salad suggestions
4 large iceberg lettuce leaves, shredded
1 tomato, chopped
1 Lebanese cucumber, diced
½ avocado, sliced
½ carrot, shredded
¼ capsicum, seeds and membrane removed, chopped
½ cup (60 g) grated cheddar
3 tablespoons tomato salsa (bought or homemade)

1. Reheat the meat sauce in a large frying pan over medium heat.
   Add the kidney beans and heat through.
2. Meanwhile, heat the taco shells following the packet instructions.
3. Fill the shells with the beef mixture and your choice of salad
   ingredients. Serve and enjoy!

ROBYN'S BAKED SALMON WITH ALMOND AND OLIVE PESTO

Serves 4

4 x 150 g salmon fillets, with or without skin
200 g green beans
250 g baby tomatoes
1 tablespoon olive oil
dill and lemon wedges, to serve

Almond and olive pesto
1 cup (160 g) almonds
½ cup (60 g) pitted green olives
½ cup roughly chopped flat-leaf parsley
3 tablespoons roughly chopped dill
2 teaspoons finely grated lemon zest
1 garlic clove, chopped
2 tablespoons olive oil

1. Preheat the oven to 200°C and line a baking tray with baking paper.
2. To make the pesto, place all the ingredients in a food processor and blitz to a chunky paste.
3. Place the salmon fillets on the prepared tray and spread 2 tablespoons pesto over each one.
4. Toss the green beans and baby tomatoes with 1 tablespoon olive oil and add to the tray with the salmon. Bake for 12–15 minutes or until just cooked through.
5. Garnish with dill and serve with lemon wedges.

Tip: Spoon the leftover pesto into a jar and cover with a thin layer of extra oil. Seal and store in the fridge for up to 2 weeks. Enjoy it as a dip with sliced carrot and celery or as a snack, spread on wholegrain toast.

Judith is an active member of the IWL community and has successfully achieved and maintained her goals. These are some of her favourite 'go to' IWL recipes.

JUDITH'S RATATOUILLE

Serves 4

1 tablespoon olive oil
1 garlic clove, finely chopped
2 brown onions, finely chopped
200 g chicken breast or lamb fillet, cut into thin strips (optional)
1 eggplant, sliced
1 zucchini, cut into bite-sized pieces
1 red or green capsicum, seeds and membrane removed, cut into
    bite-sized pieces
4 tomatoes, chopped (or use a 400 g tin chopped tomatoes)
1 bay leaf
½ teaspoon dried thyme
1 x 400 g tin chickpeas, drained and rinsed
sea salt and freshly ground black pepper

1. Heat the olive oil in a large frying pan over medium heat, add the garlic and onion and cook for 1–2 minutes or until lightly golden. Add the meat (if using), eggplant, zucchini and capsicum and cook for a few minutes or until the meat is cooked through and the vegetables begin to soften.
2. Add the tomatoes and herbs and cook until the tomato juice evaporates and thickens. Stir in the chickpeas and warm through. Season to taste with pepper and serve.

Tip: Many people like to salt the eggplant before cooking but it's not necessary because a lot of the overwhelming bitterness has been bred out of this vegetable.

JUDITH'S BEAN, TOMATO AND EGG SALAD

Serves 4

300 g green beans, cut into large bite-sized pieces
2 eggs, at room temperature
2 tomatoes, cut into bite-sized pieces
1 x 400 g tin cannellini beans, drained and rinsed
freshly ground black pepper, for seasoning

Vinaigrette
1 tablespoon olive oil
1 tablespoon red wine vinegar
1 tablespoon wholegrain mustard

1. Bring a medium saucepan of water to the boil, add the beans and cook for 3 minutes or until tender-crisp. Drain and allow to cool in refrigerator.
2. Meanwhile, cook the eggs in a small saucepan of simmering water for 7 minutes. Remove and cool, then peel and cut into large bite-sized pieces.
3. To make the vinaigrette, combine all the ingredients in a small bowl or jug.
4. Combine the tomato, cannellini beans, green beans and egg in a large bowl. Dress with the vinaigrette, season to taste with black pepper, and serve.

JUDITH'S VEGETABLE FRITTATA

Serves 4

1 cup (200 g) green lentils
olive oil spray
2 tablespoons fresh breadcrumbs
2 cups chopped mixed vegetables of all colours
4 eggs
100 g feta, roughly chopped

1. Cook the lentils according to the packet instructions.
2. Preheat the oven to 180°C. Lightly spray a medium-sized baking dish with olive oil, add the breadcrumbs and gently turn the dish so they stick to the bottom and sides. (This will prevent the eggs from sticking during cooking.)
3. Meanwhile, steam or boil the mixed vegetables until just tender.
4. Arrange the vegetables and lentils evenly in the dish, then gently pour the lightly beaten eggs over the top. Sprinkle with the feta and bake for 30 minutes or until the egg is set. Cut into four pieces and enjoy.

JUDITH'S FREEKEH, POMEGRANATE AND KALE SALAD

Serves 4

1 cup (180 g) freekeh
½ cup (100 g) green lentils
large handful of kale leaves, stems removed
1 cup coriander leaves, finely chopped
½ cup flat-leaf parsley leaves, finely chopped
3 tablespoons finely chopped mint
1 small red onion, finely chopped
2 tablespoons pistachios, roughly chopped
2 tablespoons pine nuts, lightly toasted (see Tip)
2 tablespoons baby capers
½ cup (80 g) currants (optional)

Yoghurt dressing
1 cup (280 g) natural yoghurt
1 teaspoon cumin seeds, toasted and ground
½ teaspoon ground cinnamon

Topping
seeds of 1 pomegranate
2 tablespoons pumpkin seeds
2 tablespoons slivered almonds

1. Cook the freekeh and lentils separately according to the packet instructions. Drain and set aside in a large bowl to cool.
2. Add the remaining salad ingredients to the bowl and gently toss to combine.
3. To make the dressing, whisk together all the ingredients in a bowl or jug.
4. To finish, sprinkle the pomegranate seeds over the salad and drizzle over the yoghurt dressing. Top with the pumpkin seeds and slivered almonds and serve.

Tips: If you don't have any freekeh in your cupboard, brown rice works just as well here.
To toast the pine nuts, see Tip on p. 303.

SNACKS AND SIDES

BRUSCHETTA

Bruschetta is an antipasto from Italy, traditionally consisting of grilled bread rubbed with garlic and topped with olive oil and salt. Save yourself the embarrassment of ordering it at a restaurant and inevitably mispronouncing it, and make it in the safety of your own home! This version is a favourite of ours and makes a delicious snack when entertaining guests.

Serves 4

4 slices sourdough (or your favourite bread)
250 g cherry tomatoes or 3 regular tomatoes, roughly chopped
handful of basil, roughly chopped
½ red onion, finely chopped
2 garlic cloves, crushed into a paste
1 tablespoon balsamic vinegar
freshly ground black pepper, to season

1. Lightly toast your bread with the garlic spread across the top.
2. Meanwhile, mix all the remaining ingredients in a bowl.
3. Spoon the tomato mixture over the bread, season with black pepper and serve.

BASIL AND CASHEW PESTO

This delicious pesto is far healthier than the ready-made pesto you can buy at the supermarket. If you are growing basil at home, it's even better.

Makes about 1 cup

2 cups basil leaves
1 garlic clove, crushed
⅓ cup (50 g) cashews or pine nuts, lightly toasted
⅓ cup (25 g) grated parmesan
⅓ cup (80 ml) olive oil

1. Blend the basil, garlic, nuts and parmesan in a food processor until well combined. Gradually add the olive oil in a thin stream until well combined.

Tip: Store in an airtight jar with a thin layer of olive oil across the top. This can be kept in the fridge for 2 weeks.

KALE PESTO

This is wonderful way to use up an abundance of home-grown produce. Here we use a traditional mortar and pestle for a more rustic finish, but you can of course make this in a food processor if preferred. Serve on pasta, as a dip, or with salad.

Makes about 1 cup

large bunch of kale leaves, stems removed
large bunch of basil leaves
2 garlic cloves
1 tablespoon olive oil
1¼ cups (100 g) grated parmesan
3 tablespoons pine nuts, lightly toasted (see Tip, page 303)
small handful of walnuts

1. Place all the ingredients in a mortar and mash with a pestle until you are happy with the consistency. It requires a fair bit of manual labour (see it as a good workout!) and can take up to 20 minutes.

Tip: Store in an airtight jar with a thin layer of olive oil across the top. This can be kept in the fridge for 2 weeks.

ROAST CAULIFLOWER

Roast cauliflower is perfect for entertaining – it's easy, delicious, very impressive and you can whack it in the oven and forget about it. The leaves are also edible.

3 tablespoons olive oil
1 head cauliflower, with the leaves on
juice of 1 lemon
1 tablespoon capers
2 teaspoons wholegrain mustard
freshly ground black pepper

1. Preheat the oven to 180°C and line a baking tray with baking paper.
2. Drizzle 2 tablespoons of the olive oil evenly over the cauliflower and season with pepper. Roast for 45–60 minutes or until golden and tender when tested with a knife. Start checking after 45 minutes, as the cooking time will depend on your oven.
3. Meanwhile, whisk together the lemon juice, capers, mustard and remaining olive oil.
4. Remove the cauliflower from the oven and drizzle the dressing over the top. Take the whole cauliflower to the table and let everyone cut off as much they want.

OTHER SNACKS ON THE IWL PLAN

- nuts
- seeds
- homemade dips (such as hummus or beetroot dip)
- carrot and celery sticks
- any type of oven-roasted vegetables
- fruit
- yoghurt (with no added sugar)
- boiled eggs
- wholegrain toast with 100 per cent nut spread, avocado, or 100 per cent fruit spread
- blueberries or raspberries with yoghurt

SWEET TREATS

I have deliberately excluded sweets and desserts from this book, although I do include some in the free weekly e-newsletter, if you wish to sign up, and recipes are included in the IWL online program. It really doesn't matter what you have when you bake sweet treats, as long as you are not eating them all the time. I recommend only including them once a week during the weight-loss months of the IWL plan, and twice a week on the weight-maintenance months of the plan. If you live alone, I strongly encourage you to only bake when you are going to visit friends or family, so that you can take it with you to share. Otherwise, you may find yourself at home devouring the whole lot so it doesn't go to waste.

ACKNOWLEDGEMENTS

Firstly, I'd like to thank the community of people following the *Interval Weight Loss* plan, some for many years. The continued development of this important message would not be possible without you, particularly those that have helped co-design the *Interval Weight Loss* online program, so that additional support tools are available for people to succeed on their IWL journey. A special shout out goes to Lorraine, Lynne, Judy, Tim, Aisling, Robyn, Michelle, Angus, Darlene, Fran, Megan, Joseph, Jessica, Belinda, Stephanie, Jenny, Sam and Nina.

To my wife, Sally. Thank you for always being there for me and for putting up with my fixation to change the world. Without you, I would not be able to do everything I set out to achieve. I am blessed to have such an intelligent and gorgeous person in my life. I love you very much.

To my mother, Diane, and my brother, Andrew. I am also blessed to have such a loving, helpful and kind-hearted mother and brother. All your love, support and generosity enable me to do such things as write a book. I love you both very much.

To all those people in my life who have helped shape this book – particularly Kris Klein, Ed White, Chris Wilkins and Matt Mooney. I am very thankful for all your help and truly value your friendships. This journey has been fun as we work to change the world. I would also like to thank my friends Tarley, Lenore and Nicole, who have read and edited different stages of the book.

I would like to acknowledge someone who has had a hugely positive impact on my career progression. Professor Ian Caterson has been a true mentor. He has guided me with his calm wisdom and he has encouraged me to step beyond my boundaries and to drive my ideas beyond their original scope. I would like to thank Ian for everything that he has done and continues to do, and I hope that one day I can light the path for the next generation in the same way that Ian has done for me.

Lastly, to my publisher, Penguin Random House. This is, of course, not possible without your support and belief in me, particularly Nikki Christer and Sophie Ambrose. Sophie, thank you for your wisdom and professionalism along the way. And to Genevieve Buzo, for your expertise in editing this book.

Discover a
new favourite